EASY EXERCISES

for

Aerobic Fitness

The Stay Fit Series

A Special Report published
by the editors of *Healthy Years*
in cooperation with UCLA Health

Easy Exercises for Aerobic Fitness: The Stay Fit Series

Consulting Editor: Ellen Wilson, PT, Director of Therapy Services, UCLA Health

Author: Jim Brown, PhD
Editor, Belvoir Media Group: Matthew Solan
Creative Director, Belvoir Media Group: Judi Crouse

Publisher, Belvoir Media Group: Timothy H. Cole
Executive Editor, Book Division, Belvoir Media Group: Lynn Russo

Print ISBN 978-1-879620-25-4
Digital ISBN 978-1-941937-78-5

To order additional copies of this report or for customer-service questions, please call 877-300-0253 or write: Health Special Reports,
535 Connecticut Avenue, Norwalk, CT 06854-1713. To subscribe to the monthly newsletter *Healthy Years*, call 866-343-1812
or write to the address above.

This publication is intended to provide readers with accurate and timely medical news and information. It is not intended to give personal medical advice, which should be obtained directly from a physician. We regret that we cannot respond to individual inquiries about personal health matters.

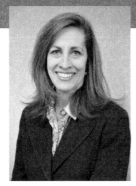

Ellen G. Wilson, PT, MS, Director, UCLA Therapy Services

If you are ready to start an exercise program, aerobic fitness is the place to begin. If you are already exercising but ready to pick up the pace, aerobic exercises and activities will improve the quality of your life and may even extend it by focusing on wellness.

Every exercise program, especially those for middle-aged and older adults, should include balance, core fitness, flexibility, strength, and most importantly, aerobic (cardiovascular) fitness.

Many of you are already using the *Special Reports in the Stay Fit Series: Easy Exercises for Balance and Mobility*, and *Easy Exercises for Core Fitness*. Now you have this report—*Easy Exercises for Aerobic Fitness*. It is filled with information, illustrations, instructions, sample programs, and the latest research used by physicians, physical therapists, exercise physiologists, and the other health professionals at UCLA Health.

What is great about an aerobic fitness program is that you'll have total control of your own exercise regime. You can begin today, exercise alone or with a group at little or no cost, and go at your own pace. You'll be able to choose from a wide variety of activities that includes walking, jogging, swimming, cycling, dancing, water exercises, aerobics classes, or simply working (or working out) at home. You can incorporate many aerobic activities into your daily routine.

We appreciate your interest in becoming or staying physically fit, and the UCLA community wants to do everything it can to make your aerobic fitness experience one that is enjoyable, productive, and long-lasting.

Sincerely,

Ellen Wilson

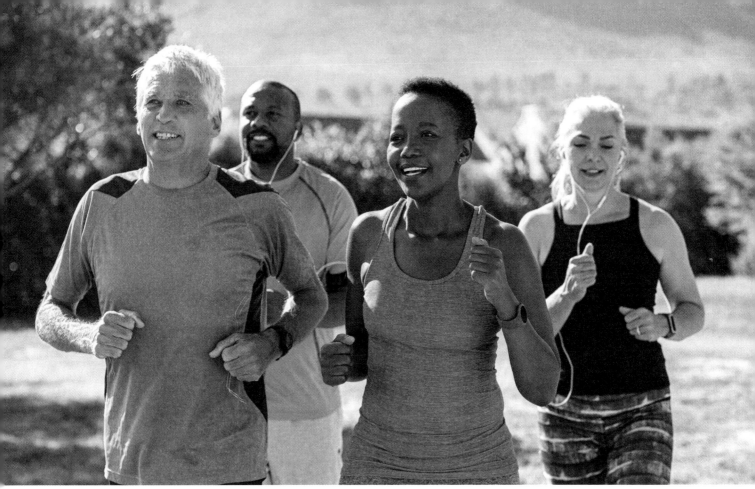

© Rido | Dreamstime

Research Findings

1

EASY EXERCISES
FOR
AEROBIC FITNESS

THE STAY FIT SERIES

A Special Report published by the editors of **HEALTHY** *Years* in conjunction with

UCLA Health

2

EASY EXERCISES
FOR
BALANCE & MOBILITY

THE STAY FIT SERIES

A Special Report published by the editors of **HEALTHY** *Years* in conjunction with

UCLA Health

3

EASY EXERCISES
FOR
BONES & JOINTS

THE STAY FIT SERIES

A Special Report published by the editors of **HEALTHY** *Years* in conjunction with

UCLA Health

4

EASY EXERCISES
FOR
CORE FITNESS

THE STAY FIT SERIES

A Special Report published by the editors of **HEALTHY** *Years* in conjunction with

UCLA Health

5

EASY EXERCISES
FOR
FLEXIBILITY

THE STAY FIT SERIES

A Special Report published by the editors of **HEALTHY** *Years* in conjunction with

UCLA Health

6

EASY EXERCISES
FOR
STRENGTH & POWER

THE STAY FIT SERIES

A Special Report published by the editors of **HEALTHY** *Years* in conjunction with

UCLA Health

7

EASY EXERCISES
FOR
MORE STRENGTH & POWER

THE STAY FIT SERIES

A Special Report published by the editors of **HEALTHY** *Years* in conjunction with

UCLA Health

8

EASY EXERCISES
10 ACTIVITIES FOR
FITNESS & FUN

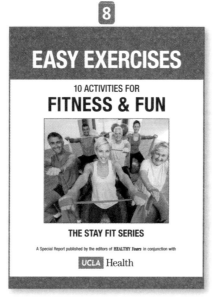

THE STAY FIT SERIES

A Special Report published by the editors of **HEALTHY** *Years* in conjunction with

UCLA Health

9

EASY EXERCISES
WALKING

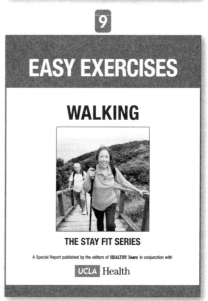

THE STAY FIT SERIES

A Special Report published by the editors of **HEALTHY** *Years* in conjunction with

UCLA Health

1. Easy Exercises for Aerobic Fitness

Cardio fitness is another term for aerobic exercise, the act of elevating your heart rate to boost cardiovascular performance and endurance. You can achieve peak aerobic fitness in a variety of heart-healthy ways. Our *Aerobic Fitness* guide describes how to safely engage in these fun and challenging activities—and explains the many ways they benefit your health.

2. Easy Exercises for Balance & Mobility

An antidote for the potentially dire result of falling down, *Easy Exercises for Balance & Mobility* describes the connection between balance and mobility, and offers exercises and specific information on how to build up crucial muscles for upper-body and lower-body strength. It also delves into the critical need for flexibility and how to achieve it without injury. Improving your balance and mobility is key to life-long independence. Just a few of these exercises a day can help.

3. Easy Exercises for Bones & Joints

As we get older, our bones and joints are not what they used to be, but we can maintain our strength and power by taking proper care of them. The key to a healthy exercise program is to get started and, then, to keep it up, making it a regular part of your life. Avoiding injury is crucial to these goals, and it often comes down to maintaining function and alleviating pain in our complex system of joints. *Bones & Joints* is intended to help you stay ahead of fitness-robbing injuries so you'll live to play again.

4. Easy Exercises for Core Fitness

Some of the most important muscles in the body are those in the hips, pelvis, abdomen, and trunk—otherwise known as "the core." And make no mistake: We use our core in every aspect of daily life. In *Core Fitness*, you'll learn the most beneficial types of core exercises and how to plan a routine, from exercises that involve free weights and dumbbells to others that use stability balls and resistance bands.

5. Easy Exercises for Flexibility

Cardio, core, and strength training, while important, don't complete the total fitness picture. Don't overlook the importance of proper warm-up and stretching, a key ingredient for better balance, and protection from injuries that can derail our quality of life. Our *Easy Exercises for Flexibility* guide describes the proper way to do static and dynamic stretching and deal with muscle soreness, as well as how to avoid injury, and more. Good flexibility is key to conducting all other exercises properly.

6. Easy Exercises for Strength & Power

Don't be intimidated by the thought of building and toning muscle. Our *Strength & Power* guide isn't about training for bodybuilding competitions. Rather, it discusses weight and resistance training for any age—always with safety first—using free weights, dumbbells, medicine and stability balls, resistance bands, weight machines, and more. Many of these exercises can be done at home as well as in a gym.

7. Easy Exercises for More Strength & Power

To maintain peak muscle efficiency, it's important to periodically advance your exercise routine. With *More Strength & Power*, you'll be able to create a program that focuses on the areas you need it most, and then change it as you progress. In this report, you'll find 55 exercises and 15 programs for your upper body, core, and lower body that will help keep you fit and in the prime of your life.

8. Easy Exercises: 10 Activities for Fitness & Fun

For some, climbing onto that treadmill and doing 30 or 45 minutes a few times a week can become a chore. Fortunately, there are myriad ways to stay fit while having fun along the way. Popular alternatives such as yoga, tai chi, qigong, water workouts, and dance are front and center in *10 Activities for Fitness & Fun*, which not only will remind you that fitness should be fun, but it just may be your inspiration.

9. Easy Exercises: Walking

There's more to walking for exercise than putting one foot in front of the other. In *Walking*, you'll learn about multiple styles—from speed walking to Nordic to walking for mindfulness—along with a surprising number of other factors, from motivation, goal-setting, and injury prevention to weather protection, road safety, proper footwear, and more.

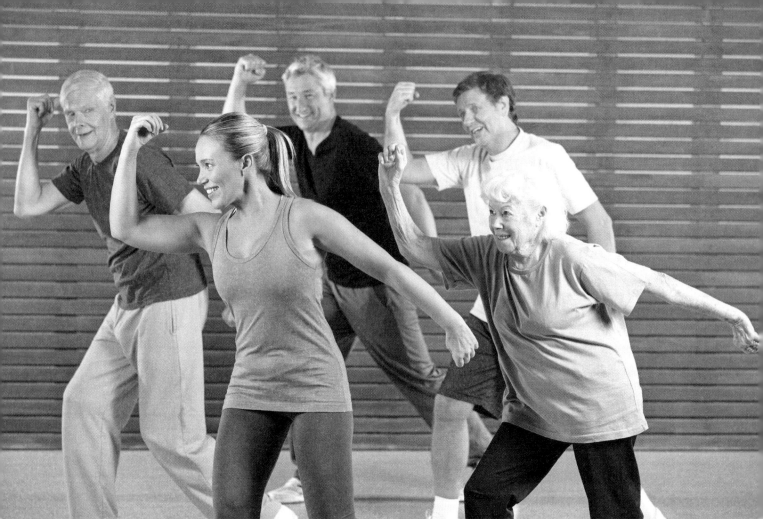

Aerobics classes are a great way to meet people and to have fun working out together.

1 Take the Aerobic Advantage

Aerobic fitness is a life-changing gift you can give yourself—one that affects every system of your body. The word "aerobic" means needing oxygen for activity, and aerobic exercise provides that oxygen.

Aerobic fitness is also called cardio-vascular fitness, which is measured two ways: 1) the amount of oxygen in blood that is pumped by the heart to the rest of the body; and 2) how efficient the body is at using that oxygen.

The way to improve aerobic fitness is through large-muscle physical activities that are demanding enough, last long enough, and are performed often enough to strengthen the heart, improve the vascular system, and increase lung capacity.

Becoming and staying aerobically fit is the most important health decision you'll ever make. No other component of fitness, whether it's strength, power, flexibility, balance, or mobility, brings with it so many added benefits.

Added Value

In addition to directly strengthening your heart, as well as increasing the efficiency of your vascular system and lungs, aerobic fitness indirectly benefits at least 10 other health-related functions, including:

1. Blood pressure
2. Cholesterol levels
3. Blood sugar
4. Stress
5. Weight
6. Disease
7. Body composition
8. Bone health
9. Mobility
10. Longevity

It Begins with Your Heart

Aerobic fitness starts with your heart. Veins carry blood to the heart, and arteries carry blood away from the heart and to the body, including the heart itself.

Your heart is a cone-shaped pump that has three layers surrounded by a fluid-filled sac. Inside, there are four chambers through which blood flows. When the valves of each chamber open and close correctly, the blood moves through the chambers and cannot back up or flow in the opposite direction. One side of the heart receives oxygen-depleted blood from the body and sends it to the lungs, where it takes on a new supply of oxygen. The other side of the heart then collects the newly-oxygenated blood and pumps it through arteries to all of the organs and cells in the body that need it to function.

Like any other organ, the heart needs oxygen to do its job, and it gets that oxygen from two big coronary arteries that carry about 5 percent of the blood supplied by the heart. When one of those arteries becomes partially blocked, it cannot supply enough oxygen-carrying blood for the heart to do its work properly. If a coronary artery becomes completely blocked, the person may have a heart attack.

What's Fitness Got To Do with It?

Exercising to become more aerobically fit makes the heart stronger, allowing it to pump more blood with each beat. The more blood pumped, the better the supply of oxygen to the rest of the body, including the heart. As a bonus, fewer beats are needed. Over time, the chamber of the heart doing the pumping (the left ventricle) adapts, gets bigger, holds more blood, and ejects more blood per beat.

A stronger heart is like having a powerful engine that can deliver oxygen

Chambers Of the Heart

Ascending aorta (to upper body)

➡ Oxygenated blood
➡ Deoxygenated blood

Aorta (to body)

Right pulmonary artery (to right lung)

Superior vena cava (from upper body)

Left pulmonary artery (to left lung)

Right pulmonary veins (from right lung)

Left atrium

Left pulmonary veins (from left lung)

Right atrium

AV

MV

PV

Left ventricle

TV

Inferior vena cava (from lower body)

Right ventricle

AV = Aortic valve
MV = Mitral valve
PV = Pulmonary valve
TV = Tricuspid valve

Descending aorta (to lower body)

© Alila07 | Dreamstime

The chambers of the heart work with the lungs to receive oxygen-poor blood, resupply with oxygen-rich blood, and pump it to the body, including the heart itself.

Pulmonary circulation system: The pulmonary circulation system involves the right side of the heart. Oxygen-depleted blood enters this side and is sent into the lungs to pick up oxygen and release carbon dioxide.

Peripheral circulation system: The peripheral circulation system uses the left side of the heart. Oxygenated blood returned from the lungs is pumped out to the rest of the body.

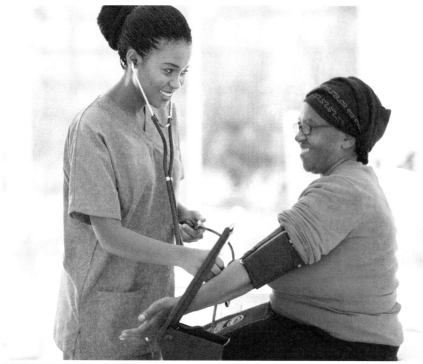
© Michaeljung | Dreamstime

Exercise can strengthen your heart, which may help lower your blood pressure.

Blood Pressure Categories

OPTIMAL BLOOD PRESSURE

Systolic ▶	Under 120 mmHg
Diastolic ▶	Under 80 mmHg

ELEVATED

Systolic ▶	120–129 mmHg
Diastolic ▶	Under 80 mmHg

STAGE 1 HYPERTENSION

Systolic ▶	130–139 mmHg
Diastolic ▶	80 – 89 mmHg

STAGE 2 HYPERTENSION

Systolic ▶	140 or more mmHg
Diastolic ▶	90 or more mmHg

HYPERTENSIVE CRISIS (EMERGENCY CARE NEEDED)

Systolic ▶	Over 180 mmHg
Diastolic ▶	Over 120 mmHg

Adapted from the American Heart Association

with greater ease. And like any other machine, the easier the workload on the heart, the longer it lasts.

Aerobic exercise also stimulates the growth of new blood vessels that supply oxygen to muscles. The result is more efficient circulation. While cardiovascular exercise increases the number of blood vessels, strength training, also called resistance training, makes them bigger.

Lower Blood Pressure

Because a stronger heart muscle can pump a greater volume of blood with less effort, less pressure is placed on the walls of arteries that distribute the blood to the rest of the body. That's why it's called blood pressure.

Blood pressure, according to the American Heart Association (AHA), is recorded as two numbers. The top number, which is always higher and called systolic, measures the pressure in arteries when the heart contracts. If too high, it is considered a major risk factor for cardiovascular disease, stroke, and other conditions among people over the age of 50. The bottom (diastolic) number reflects the pressure within arteries between heartbeats—that is, when the heart muscle is resting and refilling with blood.

The goal is to have reasonably low blood pressure, and it takes one to three months of aerobic exercise to make a difference.

A study in the journal *Hypertension* found that, for older men with high blood pressure, a brisk walk of 20-40 minutes most days of the week was enough to become moderately fit and to reduce the risk of death (see "Moderate Exercise Lowers the Risk Of Death In Men with Hypertension"). A review of 13 studies in the same publication found that hypertension could be reduced by 19 percent with four hours of exercise per week.

The normal range for adults older than 20 is lower than 120 mmHg (millimeters of mercury) for the systolic number and lower than 80 mmHg diastolic. Once your blood pressure is within the normal range, you must continue a program of aerobic fitness, combined with sensible nutrition, to keep it there. "Blood Pressure Categories" reflects blood pressure categories defined by the AHA.

Lower Blood Sugar

Exercise requires glucose, which is one of several types of sugar. Muscles and the liver release glucose to provide the fuel needed for quick bursts of activity. During longer periods of exercise the muscles get better at taking in glucose, which lowers blood sugar levels. Because one of the ways diabetes is diagnosed is by the amount of glucose in the blood, lower is better.

The amount of glucose in a person's blood changes during a 24-hour period, and there are three tests by which blood sugar levels can be diagnosed: A1C, Fasting Plasma Glucose, and the Oral Glucose Tolerance Test. The Fasting Plasma Glucose test is the one with which most people are familiar.

A normal fasting blood sugar level is between 70 and 99 milligrams per deciliter (mg/dL). "Fasting Plasma Glucose Values for Diagnosing Diabetes and Pre-Diabetes," shows the blood sugar levels for diabetes, pre-diabetes, and normal values.

Manageable Weight

According to the Centers for Disease Control and Prevention (CDC), both diet and physical activity are important in controlling weight. Most people gain weight when the amount of calories burned is less than the amount of calories taken in through food and beverages.

People vary in how much physical activity they need, so some have to be more active to maintain a healthy weight. That's where aerobic fitness comes in. The CDC says to work your way up to 150 minutes of moderate-intensity aerobic activity, or 75 minutes of vigorous-intensity, or an equivalent mix of the two each week. More about what constitutes moderate- and vigorous-intensity exercise appears later in this chapter.

To lose weight, you might need a greater amount or intensity of physical

---

Fasting Plasma Glucose Values for Diagnosing Diabetes and Prediabetes

- Diabetes: 126 or higher
- Prediabetes: 100–125
- Normal: 99 or lower

activity unless you also adjust your diet to reduce the intake of calories.

Improved Body Composition

Multiple studies have shown that aerobic exercise results in a greater increase in lean body weight, which means more muscle tissue and a lower percentage of fat tissue.

A study published in the *International Journal of Preventive Medicine* found that both light and moderate aerobics significantly improved body composition and serum lipid profiles in overweight and obese women (see "Light and Moderate Aerobic Exercise Improves Body Composition").

A study conducted at the Duke University Medical Center found that aerobic exercise is more effective for

RESEARCH FINDING

Light and Moderate Aerobic Exercise Improves Body Composition

Light and moderate-intensity aerobics significantly improved body composition in overweight and obese women, according to a study. Forty-five middle-aged women were assigned to either light aerobic exercise groups, moderate-intensity groups, or no training. The sessions lasted 10 weeks, with three 60-minute sessions per week. Both exercise groups improved in weight, fat percentage, fat weight, lean body weight, waist-to-hip ratio, and high-density lipoprotein (HDL or "good" cholesterol). The findings suggest that beginning with light aerobic exercise and advancing to moderate-intensity activity has a positive effect on multiple measures of body composition.

International Journal of Preventive Medicine

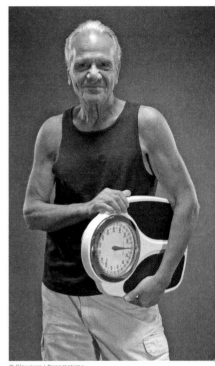

© Elswarro | Dreamstime

Keep track of your weight on a daily or weekly basis.

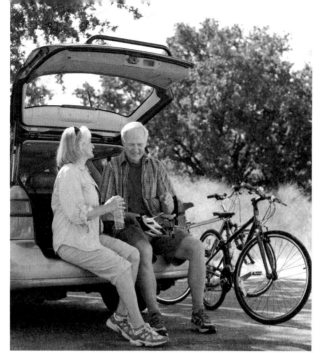

Adopting an aerobic fitness routine can help you maintain an active lifestyle.

burning fat than resistance training. And the American College of Sports Medicine acknowledges in its *Current Comment* that aerobic activities are used to improve health status, reduce disease risk, improve physical fitness, and modify body composition.

Better Mobility

Several studies have linked aerobic exercise and aerobic fitness to improved mobility. At the University of Florida, a trial with more than 1,600 older adults found that subjects in an aerobic exercise group were significantly more mobile at the end of a two-and-a-half-year monitoring period than a control group (see "Mobility Can Be Increased with Moderate-Intensity Aerobic Exercise").

RESEARCH FINDING

Mobility Can Be Increased with Moderate-Intensity Aerobic Exercise

Older adults may be able to lower their rates of disability and improve their mobility by participating in a daily moderate-intensity exercise program of aerobic, resistance, and flexibility activities. Researchers at the University of Florida assigned more than 1,600 adults between the ages of 70 and 89 to an exercise group or to a health education group, and tracked their health for an average of 2.6 years. Those in the exercise group showed significantly more mobility at the end of the period than those in the health education group, in spite of normal functional decline that occurs late in life.

Journal of the American Medical Association

The association is as much common sense as science. People who are motivated and able to follow through on a long-term exercise program are more mobile and independent than more sedentary individuals. Even those who are limited by disabilities and confined to wheelchairs can increase their mobility through aerobic-type exercises. Overcoming mobility issues also produces mental and emotional benefits.

Disease Control/Prevention

Exercise appears to help the body's immune system deal with bacterial and viral infections, according to the National Institutes of Health. The mechanism isn't clear, but there are at least four theories:

1. Physical activities may flush bacteria from the lungs and carcinogens from the body by increased output of waste through urine and perspiration.
2. Exercise pushes antibodies and white blood cells through the body at an accelerated rate, which may allow for earlier detection of illnesses.
3. The body's elevated temperature during exercise may prevent the growth of bacteria.
4. Exercise slows the release of stress-related hormones that normally increase the risk of illness.

The relationship between exercise and specific diseases varies, depending on the disease. For example, men and women who exercise 30 to 60 minutes a day have a 30 to 40 percent lower risk of developing colon cancer. The risk declines with more activity. Seventy-five to 150 minutes of exercise per week lowers the risk of breast cancer in women. Physical activity may lower the risk of lung cancer, but the evidence is not conclusive. Below are just a few of the conditions and diseases affected positively by exercise or negatively by the lack of it.

- Cardiovascular disease
- Colon cancer

- Breast tumors
- Diabetes
- Arthritis
- Parkinson's disease
- Osteoporosis
- Asthma
- Back pain
- Intestinal disorders
- Mental decline
- Emotional disorders

Two recent studies showed the effects of aerobic exercise on diabetes and Parkinson's disease, respectively. University of Iowa researchers confirmed that patients with mild to moderate symptoms of Parkinson's disease can safely participate in aerobic exercise programs and experience motor and non-motor benefits (see "Parkinson's Disease Patients Benefit from Walking, Aerobic Exercise").

In Australia, a research team found that changes in diet, resistance training, and aerobic exercise are modestly effective in inducing weight loss and lowering blood sugar levels in

Parkinson's Disease Patients Benefit from Walking, Aerobic Exercise

A study from the University of Iowa suggests that brisk walking may improve the physical and mental symptoms of patients with mild-to-moderate Parkinson's disease. Sixty people with the disease took part in sessions of walking at moderate intensity while wearing heart rate monitors three times a week, 45 minutes per session, for six months. Walking improved motor function and mood by 15 percent, attention and response control by 14 percent, fatigue by 11 percent, and increased aerobic fitness and gait speed by seven percent. The authors concluded that Parkinson's disease patients at the mild to moderate level can safely follow recommended guidelines for healthy adults, (which include 150 minutes per week of moderate intensity aerobic activity), and experience benefits.

Neurology

Diet, Resistance Training, and Aerobic Exercise Contribute To Weight Loss and Lower Blood Sugar Levels

Five Australian researchers designed a meta-analysis study to determine the effectiveness of a program of diet, resistance training, and aerobic exercise for the prevention of type 2 diabetes. They systematically reviewed the evidence in eight databases and 23 published articles and concluded that multi-component diabetes prevention interventions, including diet, resistance training, and aerobic fitness exercises, are modestly effective in inducing weight loss and improving fasting glucose levels and glucose tolerance in at-risk prediabetic adult populations.

International Journal of Behavioral Nutrition and Physical Activity

prediabetic adults (see "Diet, Resistance Training, and Aerobic Exercise Contribute To Weight Loss and Lower Blood Sugar Levels").

Lower Cholesterol

Cholesterol is a necessary fat-like substance that can be absorbed from the diet and produced by the body in the liver. However, when there is too much of it in the blood, some of the excess is deposited on artery walls, which increases the risk of heart disease.

Although researchers agree that exercise can lower cholesterol, the

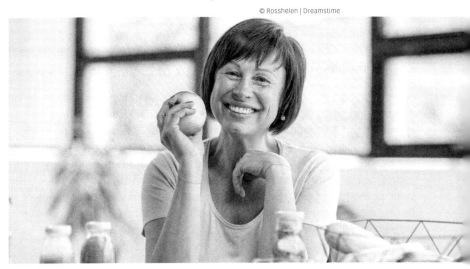

Eating healthfully can provide you with the energy you need to be active.

© Rosshelen | Dreamstime

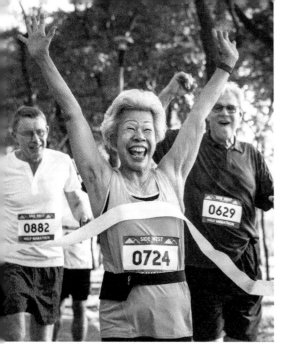
© Rawpixelimages | Dreamstime

You're never too old to achieve new goals!

mechanism by which that happens is not clear. It's possible that exercise increases the size of lipoproteins, which carry cholesterol in the blood. Small lipoproteins have been associated with an increased risk of cardiovascular disease, and some studies have shown that moderate exercise can increase their size.

Other studies suggest that exercise can improve the movement of cholesterol from the rest of the body to the liver, where it is eventually expelled. Still other investigations have shown that endurance exercise may reduce the absorption of cholesterol from the small intestine into the blood.

Perhaps the simplest theory is that losing weight results in a lower amount of low-density lipoprotein (LDL) or "bad" cholesterol in the blood. High levels of LDL is associated with heart disease.

Stress Reduction/Mood Elevation

Exercise, particularly aerobic exercise, can reduce stress by relieving tension and anxiety, serving as a diversion from daily routines, increasing energy levels, elevating mood, and improving overall emotional well-being.

Even when exercise does not change the causes of stress, it can change our perception of stress and how we respond to it. Exercise seems to force the body's systems to communicate more efficiently, according to the American Psychological Association, and this is necessary to deal with physiological and psychological stress. The more sedentary our lifestyles become, the less efficient our bodies are at responding to stress.

Lower Risk Of Fractures

The CDC says that performing aerobic and muscle-strengthening activities can slow the loss of bone density that comes with age. A study in Finland concluded that life-long physical activity in older women was associated with reduced risk of fractures. Another study, published in *Osteoporosis International*, found that exercise can reduce falls, fall-related fractures, and risk factors for falls in individuals with low bone density.

Increased Longevity

A relationship exists between moderate-intensity physical activity and longevity. *Archives of Internal Medicine* published an article a decade ago concluding that moderate levels of physical activity expanded total life expectancy, and the gains were twice as long at higher activity levels.

The Journal of the American College of Cardiology reported that leisure-time running was associated with a significantly lower risk of death (see "Leisure-Time Running Reduces the Risk Of Death from All Causes"). A study in *PLOS Medicine* found that people who engaged in leisure-time physical activity had life expectancy gains of as much as four-and-a-half years.

The CDC reports that people who are physically active for approximately four to seven hours a week have a 40 percent lower risk of dying early than those who are active for less than 30 minutes

RESEARCH FINDING

Leisure-Time Running Reduces the Risk Of Death from All Causes

Until now, little has been known about the effect of leisure-time running on the causes of death. A 15-year study of more than 55,000 adults between the ages of 18 and 100 compared the health and mortality of runners and non-runners. Runners had 30 and 40 percent lower adjusted risks of death from all causes, including cardiovascular disease, compared with the non-runners. Also, running five to 10 minutes per day at speeds slower than six miles per hour (often defined as jogging) was associated with a significantly lower risk of death. The findings may motivate healthy but sedentary individuals to begin a running program for health benefits that are sustainable throughout life.

Journal of the American College of Cardiology

Risk of Dying Prematurely Declines with Physical Activity	
HOURS PER WEEK	RELATIVE RISK
½ hour	1
1.5 hours	0.8
3.0 hours	0.73
5.5 hours	0.64
7.0 hours	0.615

Adapted from the Office of Disease Prevention and Health Promotion

a week. The risk of dying prematurely declines as you become more active. "Risk of Dying Prematurely Declines with Physical Activity," shows the relative risk, represented by the number one, and that with each increment of moderate or vigorous physical activity the risk declines.

Total Fitness Components

Although aerobic fitness may be the most important aspect of fitness and confers the greatest number of beneficial side effects, it's not the only component of fitness. Others are balance and mobility, core fitness, strength and power, and flexibility. A program of aerobic fitness should be combined with elements of each.

Balance and Mobility

As the U.S. population has aged, balance and mobility have become a more vital component of fitness. The ability to move easily and lower the risk of falls is one of the challenges of aging. A well-planned program of balance and mobility exercises fits in perfectly with a routine that includes core fitness, aerobic activities, and resistance training. Balance can be improved at any age, and *Easy Exercises for Balance and Mobility*," the first special report in this series, tells you how to do it.

Core Fitness

Core fitness is at the center, literally and figuratively, of strength and power. As you will see in "*Easy Exercises for Core Fitness*," the most important muscles are those in the hips, trunk, neck, and shoulders. Together, they are called the core, and they are involved in every aspect of daily living. Whether you are sitting or standing, you are using core muscles to maintain good posture. Core muscles are necessary for flexibility, strength, and injury prevention.

Strength and Power

Strength is the force generated when a muscle or group of muscles contracts. In practical terms, strength involves lifting, pushing, pulling, and moving, whether it's your own body or an object. Those activities are as basic as getting out of bed or up from a chair, walking to the mailbox, picking up a bag of groceries, or opening a jar.

Power is a concept closely related to strength, but with age it diminishes even faster than strength. Power is how quickly you can exert enough force to produce a certain movement.

For example, can you move an object (or your body) quickly when necessary, or does it take more time than it used to? Can you walk as fast as you once walked? Can you get up and out of a chair quickly, or it is an ordeal?

We begin to lose strength, muscle mass, and muscle efficiency at about age 30. The condition is called age-related sarcopenia. People who don't get enough exercise to offset those losses will lose 3 to 5 percent of their muscle mass every decade for the rest of their lives. The rate of loss accelerates at about age 75, but can happen during the 60s, 70s, or 80s.

The good news is that you can slow or even reverse the loss of muscle at any age. It's

A physical therapist can help you focus on the right exercises for your best health.

© Ammentorp | Dreamstime

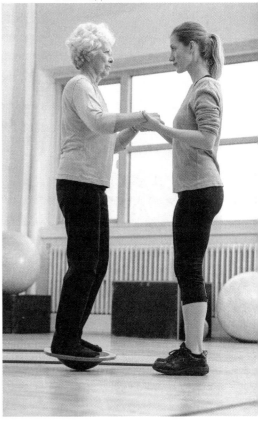

never too late. The Special Report titled *"Easy Exercises for Strength and Power"* explains and illustrates ways to increase and maintain strength and power, regardless of age.

Flexibility

Flexibility refers to the range of motion in and around a joint. Some people (and some joints) may be more flexible than others, but regardless of the person and the joint, flexibility can be improved. Among the benefits are improved range of motion and less stiffness, better balance as you get older, and improved circulation (at least temporarily). You will also be able to more easily perform activities of daily living.

Better flexibility may indirectly prevent injuries, but the evidence is not conclusive. However, regular, long-term stretching to improve flexibility might promote muscle growth, which could reduce the risk of injury. Also, exercisers who have less-than-ideal range of motion are more susceptible to muscle and joint injuries.

Stretching for flexibility is not a complete fitness package. It is not going to do much for cardiovascular fitness, and it's not going to increase muscle strength or endurance. But it remains an important component of overall fitness, and should be planned to fit your needs. For 50-plus exercises to increase flexibility, look for the special report titled *"Easy Exercises for Flexibility."*

When Does Exercise Become Aerobic?

Whatever the type of exercise, experts use terms like intensity, frequency, and duration to describe what we have to do to become or stay fit.

The basic concept of aerobic exercise (and aerobic fitness) is to exercise hard enough, long enough, and often enough to get your heart rate into a target heart zone and keep it there for a specified length of time. How intense? For how long? How often? The answers to those questions vary, depending on the source, and continue to evolve as we learn more about the body's response to exercise.

How Intense?

The "how intense?" question is answered by determining your target heart rate. Your target heart rate is your ideal heart rate while exercising. Your resting heart rate is your ideal heart rate while at rest, and your maximum heart is the rate you should not exceed for any length of time. If you are exercising and you haven't reach your target heart rate, you should increase your intensity. If you are at or above your maximum heart rate, you should slow down.

The chart to the left shows ideal target heart rates by age. However, if you prefer, you can be more specific and figure it out manually. The traditional method, according to the American Heart Association (AHA) and the American College of Sports Medicine (ACSM), is to first subtract your age from 220. That will establish your maximum heart rate.

For moderate-intensity physical activity, your target heart rate should be

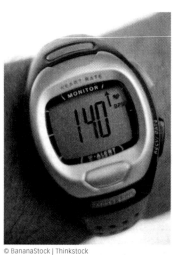
© BananaStock | Thinkstock

A heart rate monitor accurately measures your heart rate to help you stay in your target zone.

Estimated Target Heart Rate Zone By Age

AGE	TARGET 50 – 85%	AVERAGE MAXIMUM HEARTRATE 100%
20 years	100-170 beats per minute (bpm)	200 (bpm)
30 years	95-162 bpm	190 bpm
35 years	93-157 bpm	185 bpm
40 years	90-153 bpm	180 bpm
45 years	88-149 bpm	175 bpm
50 years	85-145 bpm	170 bpm
55 years	83-140 bpm	165 bpm
60 years	80-136 bpm	160 bpm
65 years	78-132 bpm	155 bpm
70 years	75-128 bpm	150 bpm

Source: American Heart Association, 2021

between 64 and 76 percent of your maximum heart rate. For vigorous-intensity physical activity, your target heart rate should be between 77 and 93 percent of your maximum heart rate.

To estimate your maximum heart rate, first subtract your age from 220. For example, for a 50-year-old person, the estimated maximum heart rate would be 170 beats per minute (bpm). So target heart rate levels would be:

64% level: 170 x 0.64 = 109 bpm
76% level: 170 x 0.76 = 129 bpm
77% level: 170 x 0.77 = 142 bpm
93% level: 170 x 0.93 = 172 bpm

Taking Your Pulse

Taking your resting heart rate is relatively easy. The best place to find your pulse is in the wrist or the side of your neck (carotid artery). But if it's easier, you can also try the inside of your elbow, or the top of your foot. To get a reading, place your index and forefinger together over the pulse site. Then using a watch or phone stopwatch app, count the number of beats you can feel within 60 seconds. Or, have someone time you while you count.

If you are sitting, or are otherwise calm and relaxed (i.e., not exercising), your heart rate should be between 60 and 100 beats per minute. If you are on a beta blocker, it is not uncommon for your heart rate to go below 60. Conversely, if you are on thyroid medication, your pulse may be slightly higher. It is nothing to worry about, but you should mention it to your doctor to be sure. Also, athletes, or people who exercise regularly every day, may also see a lower reading because their heart doesn't have to work as heart to maintain a regular steady beat.

There are other factors that can affect your heart rate, as well. For instance, if you are stressed, angry, upset, or anxious, or excited. When temperatures are extremely humid, your heart has

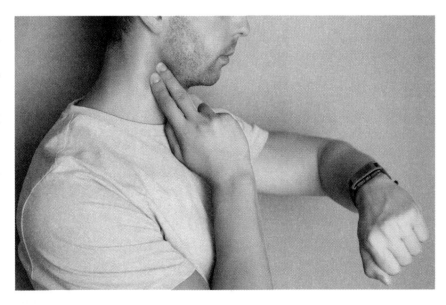

© Chernetskaya | Dreamstime

Take your pulse after exercising to ensure you are achieving your target heart rate.

© Charnsitr | Dreamstime

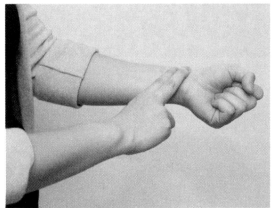

to work a little hard and your pulse rate may increase slightly. Being morbidly obese may increase your resting rate slightly because your heart has to work harder.

If you have episodes of a resting heart rate that is either too high or too low that can't be explained, or you are dizzy or you faint, call your doctor immediately.

How Long?

The ACSM recommends 20 to 60 minutes of continuous aerobic activity, but time restraints make it difficult for some people to exercise that long at one time. Now experts agree that the exercise periods can be broken down into 10-, 20-, or 30-minute sessions throughout the day. Typical moderate-intensity sessions last 20-30 minutes, not including warm-up and cool-down time.

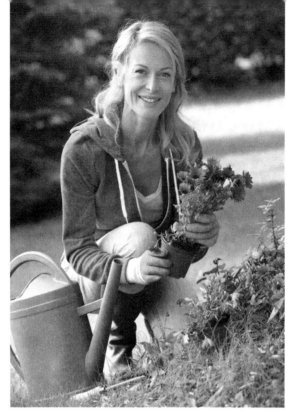

© Goodluz | Thinkstock

A moderate-intensity activity like gardening can be part of your aerobic fitness.

How Often?

The Centers for Disease Control and Prevention (CDC) recommends 150 minutes of moderate-intensity aerobic activity or 75 minutes of vigorous activity, or an equivalent mix of the two types of activity, preferably spread throughout the week—at least three times for those who exercise vigorously; five times or more for moderate-intensity workouts. An easy routine for many exercisers to follow is at least 30 minutes a day, at least five days per week.

Low-Intensity

Low-intensity exercise might be the place to start for beginners and some older adults. Something is always better than nothing. These types of exercises can get you into an exercise routine, make you more flexible, and begin to prepare your body for more demanding exercise. They also can be surprising calorie burners (see "Calories Expended Per Hour In House/Yard Chores"). Begin with low-intensity exercise, and gradually build up to a moderate-intensity level and perhaps to a high-intensity exercise program later. Examples include:

Low-Intensity Activities
- Walking leisurely
- Stretching
- Housework, yard work
- Lifting hand weights (dumbbells)
- Wall push-ups or modified push-ups

Moderate-Intensity Activities
- Walking fast
- Riding a bicycle < 10 mph
- Water aerobics
- Playing tennis (doubles)
- Mowing a lawn
- Light gardening

Vigorous-Intensity Activities
- Race walking
- Jogging/Running
- Swimming laps
- Riding a bicycle > 10 mph
- Playing tennis (singles)
- Aerobic machines/dance classes
- Heavy gardening (digging, hoeing, etc.)

Calories Expended Per Hour In House/Yard Chores

ACTIVITY	ESTIMATED CALORIES EXPENDED PER HOUR
Vacuuming	200+
Ironing	75
Scrubbing	400+
Sweeping/mopping	200–250
Carrying shopping bags	280
Grocery shopping	150
Cooking	80–100
Climbing stairs	500–600
Child care	300–600
Painting	250–300
Making beds	260
Doing laundry	150
Digging in yard	400–600
Weeding	200–230
Gardening	200–300
Car washing	150–300
Raking leaves	400–450
Mowing grass	300–350
Shoveling snow	400+

Again, the type of exercise doesn't matter, as long as you get your heart rate into the target zone and keep it there for 10 minutes or longer.

Other Ways To Measure Intensity

In addition to taking your pulse, there are other methods to determine the level of exercise. One is simply counting the number of minutes you exercise per week. The Office of Disease Prevention and Health Promotion uses total amount of aerobic physical activity as shown in "Benefits Of Total Weekly Amounts Of Aerobic Activity."

Exercise Intensity Scale

"Exercise intensity levels" start with a person at rest and progresses to an all-out sprint. It is a quick way to gauge and compare most movements or activities.

The Talk Test

The talk test is a general rule of thumb, not a highly scientific test of intensity. If you can easily carry on a full conversation and perform an activity at the same time, you probably aren't exercising aerobically, says the American Heart Association.

If you are engaged in moderate-intensity activity, you can talk but not sing while you are exercising. If you are doing vigorous-intensity exercise, you won't be able to say more than a few words

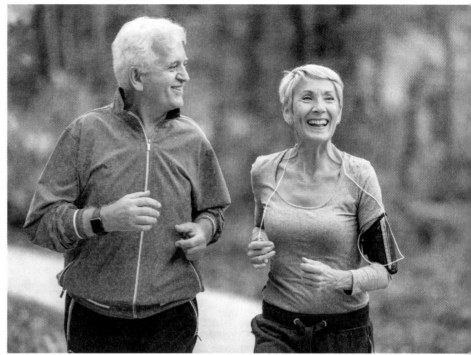

© Lordn7 | Dreamstime

without pausing for a breath. If you are out of breath or if short sentences are a strain, you are probably exercising too vigorously.

Measurement By METs

A MET (Metabolic Equivalent Task-hour) is a unit of measurement for estimating the amount of oxygen used during physical activity. One MET is equal to the amount of oxygen used at complete rest. Two-MET activities would use twice the amount of oxygen; 3-MET activities, three times the amount, etc.

If you can talk in complete sentences, speed up a little. If you can't talk at all, slow it down a bit. You should be able to say a few words but not complete sentences.

Benefits Of Total Weekly Amounts Of Aerobic Activity		
LEVEL	**WEEKLY MINUTES/ MODERATE-INTENSITY**	**OVERALL BENEFITS**
Inactive	No physical activity beyond baseline	None
Low	Activity beyond baseline but fewer than 150 minutes a week	Some
Medium	150–300 minutes a week	Substantial
High	More than 300 minutes a week	Additional

Source: Office of Disease Prevention and Health Promotion

Exercise Intensity Levels		
	0	Seated at rest
	1	
	2	Leisurely strolling
	3	
I N T E N S I T Y	4	Brisk walking
	5	
	6	Jogging
	7	
	8	Running
	9	
	10	Maximal all-out sprint

Exercise Intensity Measured By METs		
METs	**LEVEL OF EXERTION**	**ACTIVITIES**
1	Minimal	Sleeping, lying on the couch, sitting still
2	Low	Washing dishes, walking slowly, light gardening
3–6	Moderate	Golf (no cart), house cleaning, climbing stairs, cycling (10 mph or faster)
6+	Vigorous	Backpacking, high-intensity aerobics, running, tennis singles

"Exercise intensity measured by METs" gives examples of activities in terms of METs. Two-MET physical activities (walking slowly, for example) are considered low-intensity; 3-6 METs (like mowing the lawn and climbing stairs) require moderate exertion; and anything higher than six METs (like running and skipping rope) is vigorous exercise.

High-Intensity Interval Training (HIIT)

The high-intensity interval training (HIIT) movement has gained popularity among elite athletes and serious, younger, well-conditioned exercisers for several years. The American College of Sports Medicine currently ranks it as the number one fitness trend.

The science behind HIIT is that in controlled trials, short bursts of intense exercise followed by brief

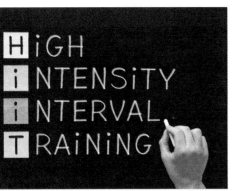

RESEARCH FINDING

High-Intensity Intervals May Improve Endurance and Lower Blood Pressure

One minute of intense exercise during a 10-minute workout three times a week increased endurance and lowered blood pressure, according to researchers at McMaster University in Ontario. Fourteen overweight men and women warmed up on stationary bicycles for two minutes, biked as hard as they could for three 20-second intervals, slow-pedaled for two minutes, and cooled down for three minutes. The authors suggested the exercise does not have to be cycling to achieve the same effects. The study represents another piece of evidence supporting the potential value of high-intensity interval training, but should not be tried without consulting a physician.

PLOS ONE

recovery breaks, repeated several times, produced the same benefits as traditional endurance training, but in much less time (usually less than 30 minutes).

Researchers at McMaster University in Canada found that just three minutes of HIIT per week improved endurance and lowered blood pressure in a group of overweight adults (see "High-Intensity Intervals May Improve Endurance and Lower Blood Pressure").

HIIT For the Rest Of Us

While HIIT seems like a good idea for the upper echelon of exercisers, there is evidence that this kind of program has value for the average person, and especially for older adults. Much of the research has been conducted on previously sedentary but otherwise healthy individuals, as well as a few studies on people with heart and metabolic diseases.

One protocol required one minute of relatively hard effort while cycling, followed by one minute of rest or light exercise, repeated 10 times, for a total of 20 minutes, three times a week. The subjects were 65 years of age or older, and had either type 2 diabetes or cardiovascular disease.

The results, published in *Medicine & Science in Sports and Exercise*, showed that the HIIT exercisers had greater improvements in cardiorespiratory fitness and reductions in blood sugar as compared to exercisers who walked the same total distance at a slower pace in a continuous manner.

Researchers in New Zealand moved their HIIT research out of the exercise laboratory and into a real-world setting—in this case, a public park program specifically designed for inactive, overweight, obese, and at-risk participants, many of whom had not exercised for years.

The results were mixed. The program produced less improvement in fitness than was seen in some laboratory-based studies. According to one of

High-intensity Interval Training (HIIT) Produces Minor Improvements In Older Adults

In Christchurch, New Zealand, researchers took their high-intensity interval training research out of the exercise laboratory and into a real world setting—a public park program for inactive, overweight, obese, and at-risk participants, many of whom had not exercised for years. The program, according to the authors, "produced less improvement in fitness than was seen in laboratory-based studies and was not the 'magic pill' hoped for, but participants did see minor improvements by the end of 12 weeks."

PLOS ONE

the authors, HIIT was not the "magic pill" they had hoped for. Yet there was some good news: Participants still experienced minor improvements by the end of the 12-week period (see "High-Intensity Interval Training (HIIT) Produces Minor Improvement In Older Adults").

Measurement Devices

Pedometers, heart rate monitors, and activity trackers are among the devices available to help exercisers keep track of their exercise intensity, duration, and frequency.

Pedometers

If you are just beginning an aerobic program, it's best to get a simple, no-frills pedometer to record the number of steps taken over a period of time or distance. Don't buy the cheapest, and don't spend a lot of money on features you probably won't use. Accurate, reliable pedometers are available for between $15 and $40. If you are ready for a more app-driven, name-brand such as Fitbit or Garmin, they run between $120 and $250, while an Apple watch starts at $150 and goes up to $400.

Features To Consider

▶ **Size:** Wrist bands generally come with two size options. A simpler pedometer fits in your pocket or attaches to a belt or waist band

▶ **Display:** Large enough to read easily in all kinds of light

▶ **Weight:** Light

▶ **Re-set button:** Automatic

▶ **Step count:** High (up to 100,000 steps)

▶ **Loss protection:** Leash or strap keeps it attached to your clothing

▶ **Extra features:** Distance and time helps determine aerobic activity

▶ **Battery life:** From months to up to 2-3 years.

The University of Illinois Wellness Center recommends a simple test to determine if a pedometer is working properly (see "Does Your Pedometer Work?").

Activity trackers provide more information than plain pedometers, although some of the projections are estimates, such as distance walked and number of calories burned. Some even record the amount of time you haven't been moving, which can be a great motivator, as well as your heart rate and your sleep patterns. In advanced models, all of the information can be uploaded to a smartphone, tablet, or desktop computer. Smartphone apps help you keep track of all the features previously mentioned and then some, like calories consumed.

Pedometers are a great way to track your distance and determine whether you are achieving your goals.

© Andrew Haddon | Dreamstime

Does Your Pedometer Work?

- Place the pedometer on your waistband.
- Set the pedometer to zero.
- Walk 50 steps.
- Read the display.

Your pedometer step count should be within four or five steps of the count you made while walking.

If not, reposition the pedometer (directly over your left or right hipbone at the midline of the thigh and directly over your knee) and try again.

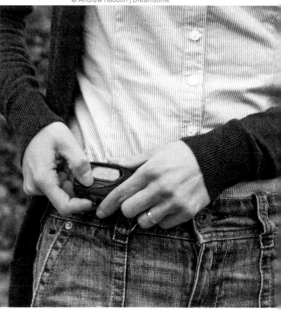

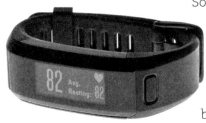

Some of the newer digital fitness trackers also monitor your heart rate.

Heart Rate Monitors

Sophisticated heart rate monitors are for heart patients whose doctors have prescribed them for medical reasons, not for the average person. A healthy person does not need to know how fast his or her heart is beating, even during exercise.

However, if you are an exerciser who wants to get more precise information about getting your target heart rate into an effective and safe zone, over-the-counter heart rate monitors may be worth the cost. According to the American College of Sports Medicine, as exercise intensity increases, oxygen consumption and heart rate increase together. Heart rate is easier to measure than oxygen consumption, and heart rate monitors accurately measure the rate.

Not surprisingly, manufacturers have gone far beyond simple counts of the heartbeat. Optional features include a watch, stopwatch, lap timer, GPS, alarm, memory, recovery rate, estimated number of calories expended, and computer links. The more features, the higher the cost—one that will count your heart rate and tell you how long you've been in the target zone will probably be in the $60 to $120 range. Once you start adding features, monitors can cost from $120 to $500, and are likely to cross the line into activity trackers rather than just heart rate monitors.

Factors To Consider
- **Types:** Chest strap (more accurate, more troublesome to wear); touch-type wristwatch (less expensive, less hassle to wear, less accurate), and continuous reading wristwatch (no chest strap, easier to read, pricier)
- **Set-up:** One that requires minimum set-up expertise and time
- **Beeper/alarm:** Sounds an alarm when your heart rate gets out of the zone, either too high for safety or too low to promote aerobic fitness

- **Display:** Big and easy to read in any kind of light
- **Extra features:** Depending on cost and how much information you want, as opposed to how much you need

Activity Trackers

The line between high-end heart rate monitors and activity trackers is thin, and continues to get narrower. Pack in the features of pedometers and heart rate monitors already mentioned, add even more functions, and you'll have an activity tracker. The most advanced models monitor your workouts, display information about your daily exercise and eating routines, and send the data to your smartphone, tablet, laptop, and desktop computer. Check phone compatibility—some apps and operating systems work only on Apple products, some only on Android phones, and some on both.

Resting Heart Rate

There are less technical ways to measure cardiovascular fitness, although they are not exact. One is resting heart rate. The principle is that the less (fewer times per minute) your heart has to beat to push oxygen-carrying blood throughout the body, the more efficient and healthy it is. A lower pulse rate, therefore, usually indicates better aerobic fitness.

Normal, healthy adults have a resting heart rate between 60 and 100 beats per minute (well-conditioned athletes may have resting heart rates in the 40s or 50s). That's a wide range with lots of individual differences and one of the reasons resting heart rate can't be the only measure of fitness.

In addition, several factors can make the heart beat faster, including physical activity, air temperature, illness, body temperature, hydration level, excitement, stress, body size, body position, and certain medications, including caffeine.

If you consistently have a heart rate higher than 100 or lower than 60, consult your doctor, especially if you have other symptoms, such as dizziness, fainting, or shortness of breath.

Heart Rate Recovery Time

Recovery heart rate refers to the time it takes your heart to return to normal after exercise. Physically fit persons have a shorter recovery time because their cardiovascular systems are more efficient, and adapt more quickly to vigorous exercise. Working with an exercise partner, follow these steps to determine your recovery time:

1. Establish your resting pulse rate.
2. Warm up, then exercise vigorously enough for two minutes to get your heart rate into its target zone.
3. Stop and have your partner take your pulse and record your heart rate.
4. Wait one minute and get a second pulse reading.
5. To get your heart rate recovery time, record the difference between the two numbers.

Now that you have your number, what does it mean? Surprisingly, there aren't many studies that tell how to interpret the results. Exercise physiologists still use the findings of a study published in *The New England Journal of Medicine* in 2001. The authors concluded that an abnormal recovery value of heart rate would be 12 beats per minute or less from the heart rate at peak exercise.

Warning/Disclaimer

If you take the heart rate recovery test and get a reading lower than 12, it does not mean you should immediately call your doctor or assume you have a cardiovascular problem.

It may, however, be one indication that your cardiovascular fitness level is less than it should be. If you are concerned, speak with your doctor and get his or her advice about beginning an aerobic fitness program, getting more information regarding your condition, or getting treatment.

Maintaining the Aerobic Advantage

Once you've reached a higher level of aerobic fitness, the idea is to maintain it by doing your 150 minutes per week of moderate-intensity activity, 75 minutes of vigorous-intensity exercise, or an equivalent mix of the two.

There is no absolute "use it or lose it" rule, but going without exercises for extended periods of time could put you right back where you started. How quickly you lose or diminish your level of fitness depends on your physical condition before stopping, and how long you stop exercising. Losing your aerobic advantage means a decreased capacity to take in, transport, and use oxygen, an increased heart rate, and possible loss of strength and flexibility.

In general, stopping an aerobic exercise program produces a significant loss of conditioning within two to six weeks, perhaps sooner. One study found that reducing physical activity for just a few days decreases function of the blood vessels in the legs, which indirectly affects overall aerobic fitness (see "A Few Days Of Inactivity Can Cause Vascular System Dysfunction").

People with low to moderate aerobic capacity show little effect of detraining during the first three weeks. But VO2 max (the maximum amount of oxygen you can utilize during intense exercise) declines to untrained levels after several additional weeks. Anecdotal reports from older adults say that the detraining effect occurs much faster. For most exercisers, resuming a training program within six weeks may restore previous levels of fitness in less time than people who started from an untrained level.

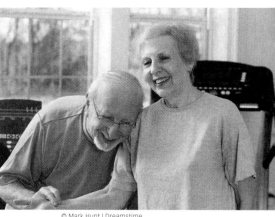

© Mark Hunt | Dreamstime

The more physically fit you are, the more quickly your heart rate returns to normal after exercise.

RESEARCH FINDING

A Few Days Of Inactivity Can Cause Vascular System Dysfunction

University of Missouri researchers found that reducing physical activity for even a few days leads to decreases in the function of blood vessels in the legs, and can take a prolonged period of time to repair. Vascular dysfunction induced by five days of inactivity required more than one day of returning to physical activity and taking at least 10,000 steps a day to improve.

Medicine and Science in Sports and Exercise

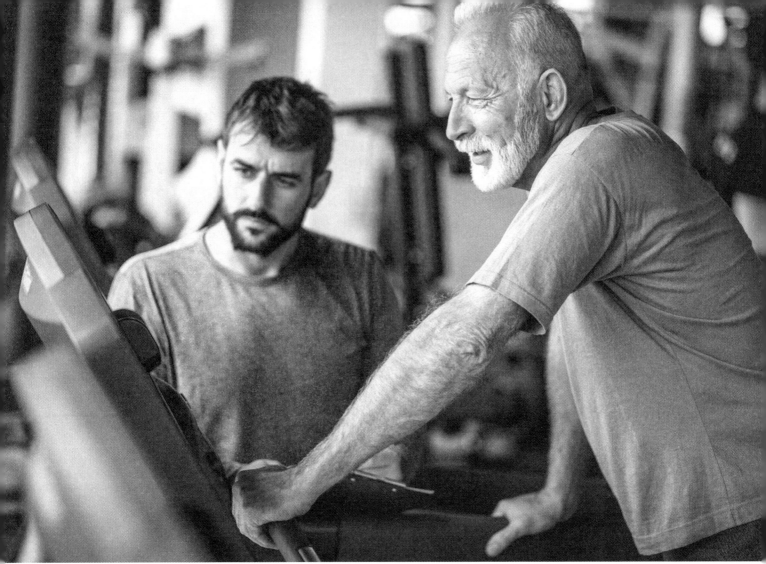

Don't be afraid to ask questions about all the bells and whistles on gym equipment. The staff are there to help you!

2 Get Ready To Go

Whatever your physical condition, regardless of age and pre-existing medical conditions, there is an exercise program out there that your doctor will approve. It may not be an aerobic exercise program at first, but any kind of exercise program—remember, something is better than nothing—will gradually put you on a path that will make you stronger, more flexible, less likely to lose your balance and fall, and have a heart and lungs that are in better shape.

For most people, starting a new exercise program with an aerobic component is safe, but first check with your doctor. If you have a specific condition(s), he or she may advise against certain types of exercises, or recommend a modified program that takes into account your specific needs and limitations (see "Conditions That May Interfere with Exercise," on page 25).

Seven Questions

The list of conditions is intimidating, even discouraging, but the Canadian Society for Exercise Physiology has developed a simple, seven-item questionnaire to help you identify health concerns that exercise might adversely affect. If you answer "yes" to any of the questions below, get medical clearance from your doctor before you begin an exercise program.

1. Has your physician ever said you have a heart condition and should only do physical activity recommended by a doctor?

2. Do you feel pain in your chest when you do physical activity?

3. In the past month, have you had chest pain when you were not doing physical activity?

4. Do you lose your balance because of dizziness, or do you ever lose consciousness?

5. Do you have a bone or joint problem (for example, back, knee, or hip) that could be made worse by a change in your physical activity?

6. Is your doctor currently prescribing drugs for your blood pressure or heart condition?

7. Do you know of any other reason why you should not do physical activity?

During your visit with your doctor, ask how often you can exercise, what types of exercise to do or to avoid, if there are any special instructions about the medications you take, and if there are steps you should take while exercising, such as checking your pulse. If you want to try a group workout or class, you might get a recommendation about where and with whom to exercise.

Play It Safe

Now that you have received medical clearance, there are some ways to exercise aerobically and safely at the same time.

If you are beginning a program, the first rule is to pace yourself. Start slowly by exercising at a pace and for an amount of time with which you are comfortable. It might be a five- or 10-minute walk, once or twice a day, two or three days a week. Once you've established a pattern of exercising, increase the time to 30 minutes or more a day, four to five days a week.

10 Percent Rule

In strength training, there is a 10 percent rule: Never increase the intensity, frequency, or duration of an exercise more than 10 percent of the previous week's

Conditions That May Interfere with Exercise

Some conditions could present health risks when exercising, according to the University of Maryland Medical Center. Check with your doctor before beginning an aerobic exercise program if you have any of the following:

- Arthritis of the hips or knees
- Blood clots
- Cardiovascular disease
- Chest pain
- Chronic lung disease
- Diabetes
- Eye injuries, recent eye surgery
- Foot/ankle sores that won't heal
- Heart disease
- Heart palpitations
- Hernia
- Hypertension
- History of smoking
- Infections
- Pain or trouble walking after a fall
- Shortness of breath

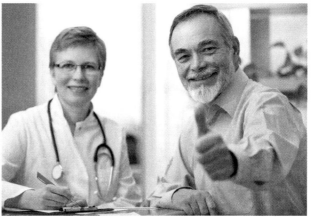

© AlexRaths | Thinkstock

Consult with your doctor to determine if it is safe to engage in aerobic activities.

workout. Aerobic exercisers might use the same rule for determining how much more they should do as they gradually make their programs more of a challenge.

In the case of walking, cycling, and swimming, for example, the time spent exercising is more important than the distance. If you can keep your heart in that target heart rate zone for 30 minutes or more at least five days a week, the distance traveled doesn't matter. However, it does give some people a sense of satisfaction knowing they have covered a certain distance.

You do not have to do the same routine for the same amount of time or same distance every day. Mixing long-exercise days with short-exercise days is okay. So is mixing types of aerobic activities or alternating exercise days with strength, flexibility, and balance/mobility workouts. Just keep in mind it's important to do something aerobically at least 30 minutes a day, five days a week.

Find An Exercise Match

The drop-out rate for exercise programs ranges from 20 to 50 percent within six months, depending on the population being studied. A study in the *Journal of Osteoporosis* found that 21 percent of exercise group participants drop out, and 16 percent of control group (no formal exercise program) participants drop out, while another 24 percent do not fully comply with the exercise parameters.

One way to ensure that you will continue with an exercise program is to find one that is a good match physically and emotionally. Ask yourself these questions:

1. Is It Age-Appropriate?

Example: Golf and bowling (even though making them a form of constant aerobic exercise may be a challenge) are sports that can be played for a lifetime. Team sports seldom are. Other sports are more suited for younger bodies.

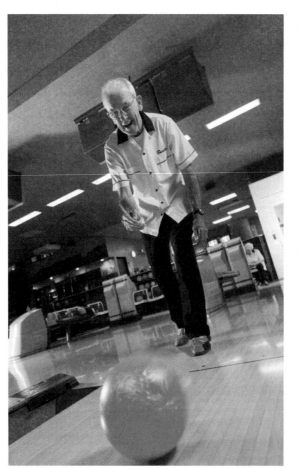

A sport like bowling can be enjoyed for a lifetime and is ideal for aging adults.

2. Does It Match Your Medical Condition?

Example: If you are obese, jogging will be a challenge. Mild-to-moderate aerobic exercises and/or dance might. If you have an orthopaedic condition (knee arthritis, for example) that could be made worse by the high-impact factor (like jogging), consider instead low-impact activities like cycling or swimming.

3. Does It Match Your Personality?

Example: If you prefer to exercise in the company of others, swimming laps is not a good match. An aerobic exercise group or walking with another person might be a better choice. If you are competitive, find an activity or sport that allows you to participate with or against others. If not, walking, jogging, and swimming provide an aerobic advantage minus the competition factor.

4. Will You Make Time?

Example: Playing a round of golf takes about four hours. If you don't have that much time on a regular basis, golf is not a good fit. Racket sports generally take less time, and walking, jogging, swimming, and aerobic exercise programs can be timed exactly to fit your schedule as long as you meet the minimum requirements.

5. Is it fun?

Example: The research is clear about this one. People stay with programs that they enjoy or from which they get satisfaction. If you dread working out, chances are you won't continue to do it. If you can make it for six months, you have a good chance of continuing for a lifetime.

6. Can you afford it?

Example: Pay-as-you-go exercise programs are great, but not if you can't afford them. Trained instructors, round-the-clock hours, and state-of-the-art equipment can be a strain on your budget. Walking and exercising at home, on the other hand, are free. City or county recreation departments, senior centers, hospitals, and YMCAs/YWCAs offer free or low-cost programs. Some low-cost programs are even covered by Medicare and insurance providers.

Plan It

One of the most common mistakes made by beginning exercisers is not scheduling workouts. You won't find time unless you make time—and not just a mental note. Add workout time to your calendar, smartphone, daily planner, or wherever you keep a schedule of other daily or weekly events. Treat it with the same importance as a meeting or lunch with a friend. It's okay to miss a day, but get right back into the schedule as soon as possible. (See the back of this Special Report for a sample two-week exercise workbook.)

Set Realistic Goals

There is a saying among management experts: "What gets measured gets done." A study in *Current Gerontology and Geriatrics Research* found that goal setting, exercise contracts, instructor feedback, self-monitoring, and exercise prompts help older adults adhere to an exercise program.

The message here is to write it down. Commit to it on paper, on your computer or in your smartphone, then check off each goal accomplished on a daily, weekly, or monthly basis. Note that branded fitness trackers, such as a Fitbit, set a basic goal of 10,000 steps a day, and will reward you when you achieve your daily goal. If the default goal is too high to start, you can manually reset your daily goal. It's better to achieve a lower goal every day than to not achieve a higher goal.

The types of goals set depend on the individual exerciser. Some people

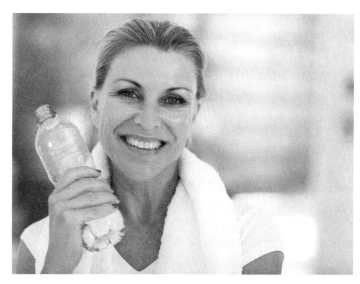

© michaeljung | Thinkstock

Drinking enough water before, during, and after exercise prevents dehydration.

respond better to long-term objectives, while others do better with week-to-week goals, gradually building up to a long-term habit of aerobic exercise.

Realistic goals for beginners or older adults might be as simple as walking, cycling, swimming, or doing aerobic exercises three days per week, 10 minutes a day, then 10 minutes twice a day, and then 10 minutes, three times a day for three to four days per week. If you can do that, you can probably increase the duration and frequency the second, third, and fourth weeks.

Stay Hydrated

The Academy of Nutrition and Dietetics (AND) says the overall goal of hydration is to minimize dehydration without over-drinking. The amount of fluids needed varies from person to person, but there are several ways to monitor your hydration status.

One is the color of your urine. Dark-colored urine (the approximate color of apple juice) is an indication of dehydration. Straw-colored or lemonade-colored urine usually means appropriate hydration.

The other is the amount of sweat lost, but this is not usually a concern for beginning or moderate aerobic exercisers. Among serious, vigorous exercisers, factors such as thirst, urine color,

- Thirst
- Flushed skin
- Fatigue
- Increased body temperature
- Faster breathing
- Faster pulse rate
- Increased perception of effort
- Decreased exercise capacity
- Dizziness
- Weakness
- Difficulty breathing during exercise

It's a good idea to keep a healthy snack, such as an energy bar, handy for after you exercise, but be sure to choose one without sodium, added sugars, or saturated fats.

© Photographerlondon | Dreamstime

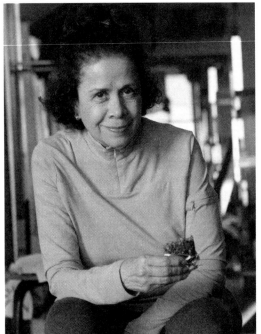

fluid intake, sweat loss, and body weight changes are taken into consideration.

What is important to remember is that dehydration can happen to anyone, any time, at any age, and under almost any circumstances—hot weather, cold weather, at higher altitudes, in the water or out, and even around the house. People in the age 50 and older group are notoriously under-hydrated. "Check Dehydration Warning Signs" gives the warning signs of dehydration for those that relate to you.

Water remains the best way to replace fluids during exercise. Drinking water rehydrates your body and cools it from the inside-out. Leave the sports drinks for those who participate in moderate to high-intensity exercise.

The American College of Sports Medicine recommends the following amount of fluid before, during, and after exercise:

- 2-3 cups of water during the two to three hours before a workout
- ½-1 cup of water every 15 to 20 minutes during a workout
- 2-3 cups of water after your workout for every pound of weight lost (if any) during a workout

Eat Right

What you eat and when you eat also affects how you feel during exercise. For beginners and older adults who may not exercise at an intense level, the rules are more flexible and should be based on what types of foods each person tolerates.

Three organizations—the American College of Sports Medicine, the Mayo Clinic, and the American Heart Association—give the following suggestions:

▶ **Before mild-to-moderate exercise:** Whole-grain cereals, bread, juices, water, coffee with breakfast, fat-free yogurt, pancakes, waffles, fruits, vegetables

▶ **Before strenuous exercise**
- Large meals at least three to four hours before
- Small meals (more than a snack) at least two to three hours before
- Snacks (apples, bananas) an hour before

▶ **After strenuous exercise:** Whole-grain English muffins, bagels, crackers, low-fat chocolate milk, juice-water blend, energy bars, low-fat granola bars, yogurt, fruits, fruit smoothies, vegetables, peanut butter sandwiches, pretzels, pasta

▶ **Note:** If weight loss is one of your exercise goals, consult with your physician or dietician to develop a meal plan to support both exercise and weight loss.

What To Wear

Choosing exercise apparel has to take into account comfort, function, style, and cost, though not necessarily in that order. If your aerobic exercise is going to take place outdoors, the weather may be the most important consideration.

Fit It

Aerobic exercise involves repetitive movement, so the first rule is to avoid any kind of fabric that is going to chafe, irritate, ride up, or slide down. Choose tops and bottoms that let you move and that don't get in the way of what you are doing. Baggy pants, for example, can get caught up in bicycle gear. Items that have a small amount of spandex (10 percent) allow for movement without being skin-tight.

Wick It

When you sweat during aerobic exercise, the layer of clothes in closest contact with your skin should draw (wick)

the moisture away and to the surface or another layer of apparel, where it can evaporate.

Nylon and polyester-blend fabrics serve that purpose. They keep you warm during cold weather, and allow you to be relatively cool in hot weather. Some fabrics have a chemical finish to enhance performance. These "performance fabrics" are available in pants, shirts, hats, shorts, underwear, and bras.

Cotton is noticeably more comfortable at first, but it absorbs perspiration, traps it, weighs the garment down, and makes it cling to your skin. During cold months, damp clothes keep you cold. There is an argument for wearing a comfortable cotton T-shirt or top during light exercise, but light exercise is not likely to put you into the aerobic exercise category.

Layer It

Dress for a temperature that is 10 degrees warmer than the outside thermometer reads. Exercise increases lots of body functions—circulation, perspiration, blood pressure, heart rate, and body temperature.

Choose exercise apparel that you can wear in layers, depending on the outside temperature or temperature of the room. Some experts tell us to think in terms of three layers: 1) a wicking T-shirt or top, 2) a warmer pullover, and 3) a protective shell or windbreaker on the outside.

Like It

Style is not high on everyone's list, but common sense says that if a person is not comfortable with the way something looks, he or she is less likely to exercise in it. Wear workout clothes you like and that motivate you.

Protect It

If you are going to exercise outside at dusk, at night, or early in the morning, wear reflective material so you can be seen (and not hit) by drivers and cyclists.

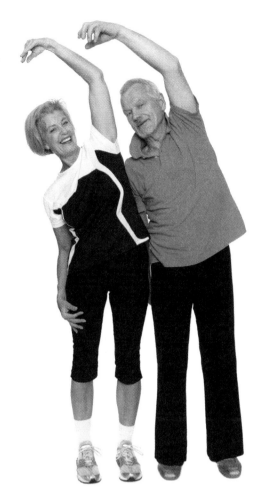

© Lammeyer | Thinkstock

Comfortable and functional clothing protects your body and makes workouts more enjoyable.

Protect your head, face, and neck. Insulate them during cold weather; shield your skin from the sun year-round with a minimum 30 SPF (sun protection factor) sunscreen.

Shoes

If playing a sport is your way to exercise aerobically, and if you play that sport more than three times a week, you should wear a sport-specific shoe (tennis shoes, for example). If not, shoes designed for aerobics or cross-training shoes should be okay.

That's the combined advice of two orthopaedic medical organizations—The American Academy of Orthopaedic Surgeons (AAOS) and the American Orthopaedic Foot and Ankle Society (AOFAS). "Shoe Features" lists specific recommendations regarding

Shoe Features	
Purpose of Shoe	**Features**
Aerobic Exercise	• Lightweight • Good shock absorption under the ball of the foot
Cross-training	• Flexible in the forefoot for running • Lateral support for aerobic exercises
Walking	• Light weight • Extra shock absorption in the heel and under the ball of the foot • Slightly rounded sole
Running	• Adequate shock absorption • Good heel control
Tennis	• Lateral support for side-to-side movement • Forefoot flexibility • Slightly less shock absorption • Softer soles for soft courts • Greater tread for hard courts

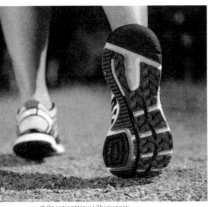
© Boarding1Now | Thinkstock

Invest in good quality shoes that are appropriate for your aerobic activity.

shoe features for different activities, and "Shoe Fitting Facts" offers suggestions on buying athletic shoes.

Problems

If you have problems with comfort, consider heel cups, arch supports, or metatarsal pads. A cup may relieve pain in the heel caused by plantar fasciitis (see page 43). Arch supports may do the same for pain in the arches, and metatarsal pads can help relieve pain and pressure beneath the ball of the big toe or the other toes.

Running shoes should be replaced after 350 to 400 miles of use, but a better way to check is to see if the back of the soles are worn out. If the shoes are giving less support, or growing uncomfortable, you may not know until you compare them to a new pair. With regular use, the general rule of thumb is to replace shoes every six months.

Socks

Often an afterthought, socks are as important as shoes for regular exercisers. Fit, durability, length, cushioning, material, and moisture management are worth mentioning.

Fit/Height

Avoid socks that are too tight or too loose. Too-tight socks may constrict the toes; too-loose socks can wrinkle, pinch, and cause blisters. Some people prefer crew-length; others like mid-calf length, and some go for knee-length socks. The most important feature is a sock that rises above the back of the shoe to prevent blisters. Don't buy socks that are shorter than the shoe.

Cushioning

A dense weave provides more padding, which can be helpful at the heel and ball of the foot. A cushioned heel may also last longer. Be careful about overly cushioned socks. They may make the shoes fit too tightly.

Material

"Moisture management" sounds a bit technical, but the one area sock experts agree on is that they should have a wicking property to draw moisture (sweat) away from the foot so it can evaporate.

Stay away from cotton athletic socks. Instead, look for synthetic fibers such as CoolMax®, DryMax®, acrylic, nylon, and polypropylene. One natural fiber called merino wool (Smartwool®) is popular in athletic socks. Socks made with polypropylene will shrink in a dryer, so drip-drying is better. CoolMax® socks are supposed to be shrink resistant.

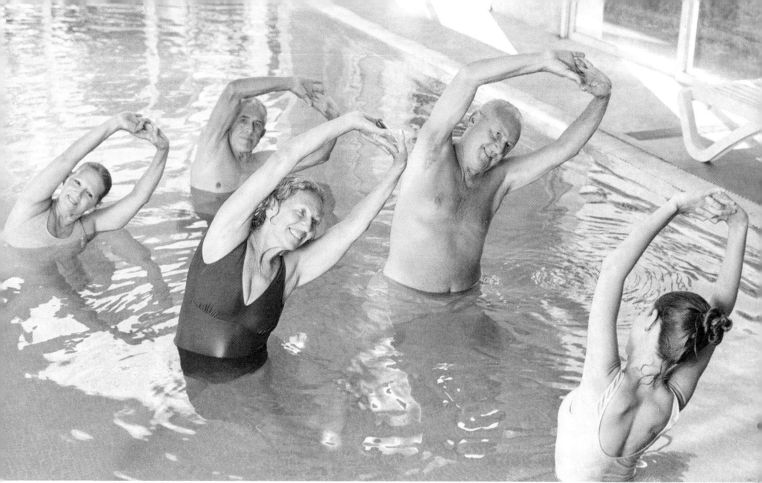

© Stylephotographs | Getty Images

3 Choose the Right Program

There is not a "one-size-fits-all" program of aerobic fitness. Instead, dozens of methods and combinations of methods have been proven effective.

The key is to find a program that works for you, one that takes into consideration your age, health status, physical condition, personality, fitness goals, and living circumstances. This chapter discusses the most popular forms of aerobic fitness programs and helps you choose the best fit. If you try one and don't like it, try another, or try a combination of physical activities that help you get into that magic target heart rate zone, and sustain it for 20 to 30 minutes.

Where To Find A Program

Finding these programs shouldn't be a problem. Most of them can be done at home or in your neighborhood. They are available in almost every format imaginable, including print, television, websites, videos, and smartphone apps. Commercial programs have names like Jazzercise, Zumba, Silver Sneakers, and Cardio Tennis. Non-profit organizations like the Arthritis Foundation and American Heart Association, as well as government agencies (Veterans Administration, the Centers for Disease Control and Prevention, and the National Institutes of Health) all offer programs.

If you prefer exercising with others, and with the supervision of a trained exercise instructor, here are some places where you might find programs.

- Local/regional hospitals
- YMCAs/YWCAs
- Churches/synagogues
- Fitness/wellness centers, gyms
- Physical therapy clinics/facilities
- Municipal recreation centers
- Senior/community centers
- Colleges/universities
- Workplace wellness centers

Exercising in water is a great way to take pressure off sensitive bones and joints, such as the knees, hips, and spine.

Easy Exercises for Aerobic Fitness | 31

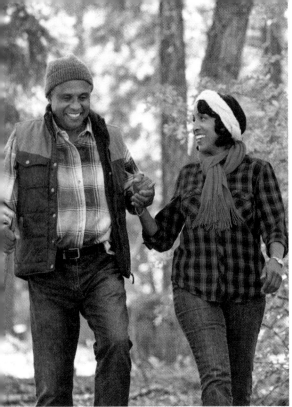

© Monkeybusinessimages | Dreamstime

Walking offers something for everyone—fresh air, companionship, scenery, and fun!

Walking

Of all aerobic activities, walking is the most natural, convenient, inexpensive, and probably the safest. If you decide to start walking for exercise, you won't be alone. Exercise walking is the number-one form of physical activity in the U.S., with more than 93 million people reporting that they walk for exercise at least once a year—not exactly a commitment to aerobic fitness, but it's a start.

Turning an occasional activity into an aerobic exercise is simply a matter of walking more often, faster, and for periods of time that eventually add up to 30 minutes or more a day, at least five days a week.

Walking is also the easiest way for a previously sedentary individual to get started on an aerobic exercise program.

Walking at the right pace and length of time can provide the same kinds of benefits bestowed by other, more rigorous activities. A study involving thousands of subjects of all ages found that brisk walking can lower the risk of cardiovascular conditions as much as running (see "Moderate-intensity Walking Can Lower the Risk Of Heart Conditions As Much As Running").

Previous studies have linked walking with improved energy, sleep, flexibility, posture, skin, and memory, lower cancer risks, better weight control, and even increased creativity (see "Walking Improves Creative Output By 60 Percent").

How Fast? How Far?

The average speed for fitness walking is between 3.0 and 3.5 miles per hour, but the pace depends on the person's age, gender, and fitness level, as well as terrain. As with other aerobic activities, the pace and distance are not as important as getting your heart rate into the target heart rate zone and keeping it there for 20 to 30 minutes at a time (three 10-minute walks per day, two 15-minute walks, or one 30-minute walk, plus warm-up and cool-down times).

Step-By-Step

The 10,000 steps program has been successful in motivating millions of people to walk. Ten thousand steps a day is about five miles, although the number of steps is based more on a

RESEARCH FINDING

Moderate-Intensity Walking Can Lower the Risk Of Heart Conditions As Much As Running

Walking briskly can lower the risk of heart-related conditions as much as running, according to the results of two studies involving more than 33,000 runners and 15,000 walkers between the ages of 18 and 80. The same energy used for moderate-intensity walking and vigorous-intensity running resulted in similar reductions in risk for hypertension, high cholesterol, diabetes, and possibly coronary disease over the six-year study period. The authors emphasized that the more runners ran and the more walkers walked, the greater the health benefits for both groups. They added that walking may be a more sustainable activity for some people when compared with running.

Arteriosclerosis, Thrombosis, and Vascular Biology

RESEARCH FINDING

Walking Improves Creative Output By 60 Percent

A study at Stanford University found that creative output increased by an average of 60 percent when people walked compared to when they sat. The researchers used four experiments with 176 people who completed tasks used to gauge creative thinking. The participants were placed in different conditions—walking indoors, outdoors, on treadmills, and sitting. The overwhelming majority in three of the experiments was more creative while walking than sitting, while 100 percent of the walking subjects in the fourth experiment displayed enhanced creative output when compared to those seated. The authors did not say that every task should be done while simultaneously walking, but those who require a fresh perspective or new ideas would benefit from it.

Journal of Experimental Psychology: Learning, Memory, and Cognition

number people can remember. It seems to work—all you need is a pedometer and some good walking shoes to get started. Remember: Walking shoes should be light, flexible at the base of the toes, and have extra shock absorption in the heel and under the ball of the foot.

First, determine your usual activity level. The American College of Sports Medicine (ACSM) suggests that you wear a pedometer for a week without altering your routine. Use "Activity Level By Daily Steps," to classify your current activity level.

According to *The Walking Site*, if you average 3,000 steps per day now, your goal for the first week should be 3,500 each day. The goal for the second week is 4,000 steps each day. Continue to increase the total each week and you should average 10,000 steps a day by the end of 14 weeks.

Ten thousand steps, although an admirable goal, may not be practical or possible for some people. At least one ACSM expert suggests that 7,500 steps may be a more reasonable number, and adds that the goal of 150 minutes of activity per week is consistent with most fitness guidelines.

Adding Steps

Try increasing the number of steps you take each day.

- Take a walk with a friend or family member
- Walk the dog
- Use stairs instead of elevators
- Park farther from stores
- Plan walking (instead of sitting) meetings
- Take walking breaks at work
- Walk to local businesses instead of driving

Hot Spots and Remedies

Although the risk of injury while walking is low, it exists. The most common injuries are blisters, shin splints, and muscle cramps. Wear cushioned and supportive shoes and socks (see page 30). Keep your feet as dry as possible, and be sure your shoes are not rubbing against any part of your foot. Try not to walk on concrete sidewalks, at least not at first. Instead, begin on asphalt, a track, or hard/wet sand, all of which are softer. At the beginning of your new walking program, stay on flat surfaces and gradually work up to hills.

Jogging/Running

These two activities are often paired together, but they are different. Jogging is often defined as moving at a speed slower than 6 miles per hour, while running is any speed faster than that. Which one you choose to do depends on your fitness level and ability. Many older adults often begin with jogging and gradually progress to running. Both activities offer all of the advantages of walking, but at a higher intensity level. Their benefits are well documented, and for many people it takes as little as 10 minutes a day to get positive health results. Like walking, all you need is time, a place to jog or run, and a good pair of well-fitted running shoes.

Jogging And Running Versus Walking

Jogging and running gives you two advantages over walking. The first is that it allows you to expend energy in a shorter period of time. Simply stated, it takes longer to walk a mile than to run or jog one. Running for 20 to 30 minutes is the equivalent to walking 40 to 50 minutes. For younger adults, brisk walking may not raise the heart rate into an optimal training zone. That's not usually a problem with middle-aged and older adults.

One of the most compelling arguments for jogging came in the Copenhagen City Heart Study, which found that joggers had a five- to six-year longer life

Activity Level By Daily Steps	
NUMBER OF STEPS	**ACTIVITY LEVEL**
0-4,999	Sedentary
5,000-7,499	Low active
7,500-9,999	Somewhat active
10,000-12,500	Active
12,500 or more	Highly active

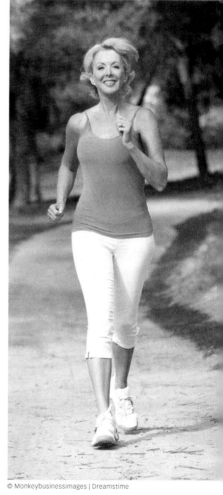

© Monkeybusinessimages | Dreamstime

Studies show that just 10 minutes of running or jogging offers many health benefits.

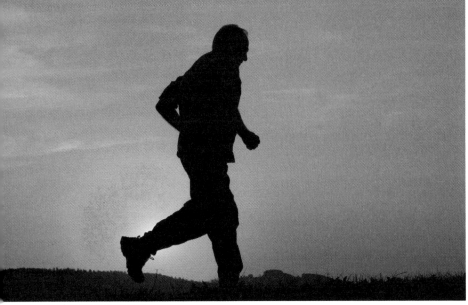

© Stefanschurr226 | Dreamstime

Joggers have a longer life expectancy than the average population.

expectancy than the average population (see "Joggers Have A Longer Life Expectancy Than the Average Population").

Another study found that seniors who jog regularly walk as efficiently as younger adults (see "Jogging Helps Older Adults Walk More Efficiently").

Jogging and running are high-impact exercises, as opposed to low-impact (one foot always on the ground) activities, and they require a higher degree of dedication. One study showed that 50 percent of people who begin a jogging/running program drop out, compared to 20 percent of those in a walking program.

Risks

With the added advantages of jogging come risks. Joggers and runners have a higher risk of injuries than walkers, and the risk increases with the frequency and duration of running. Every time a jogger's foot hits the ground, the impact is three to four times his or her body weight, as compared to the surface impact of walking. One study showed that as many as 66 percent of joggers and runners sustain an injury during a one-year period.

Hot Spots and Remedies

The most common running injuries are shin splints, plantar fasciitis, cramps, neck and back pain, and blisters. UCLA physical therapists recommend a dynamic warm up and static stretching cool down as part of a jogging/running program that focuses on calves,

RESEARCH FINDING

Joggers Have A Longer Life Expectancy Than the Average Population

The Copenhagen City Heart Study of more than 17,000 healthy men and women between the ages of 20 and 98 found that jogging was associated with a significantly lower all-cause mortality rate, and a substantial increase in survival rates for both men and women. The findings showed that between one and two-and-a-half hours of jogging per week at a slow or average pace delivered the greatest benefits for longevity. Life expectancy of men was increased by more than six years, and more than five years for women. According to the authors, "We can say with certainty that regular jogging increases longevity. The good news is that you don't actually need to do that much to reap the benefits."

Arteriosclerosis, Thrombosis, and Vascular Biology

RESEARCH FINDING

Jogging Helps Older Adults Walk More Efficiently

A study conducted by researchers at the University of Colorado and Humboldt State University found that seniors who jog regularly walk as efficiently as young adults. The study involved 30 volunteers, average age 69, who had either walked or jogged 30 minutes a day, at least three days a week, for at least six months. Testing for walking efficiency showed that those in the jogging group were seven to 10 percent more efficient at walking than older, sedentary adults, as well as older adults who walked regularly as their primary form of exercise. Decline in walking ability is a predictor of morbidity in seniors. Not only did jogging improve walking efficiency, but joggers' metabolic cost of walking (the amount of energy consumed) was similar to that of young adults in their 20s, and they were less likely to experience age-related physical decline in walking efficiency.

PLOS ONE

hamstrings, quadriceps, and core (see pages 52 and 53 for static stretching exercises that address these areas.)

From Walking to Jogging

If you decide to embark on a jogging or running program, work into it gradually. Begin with a basic, but challenging, walking program, then progress to a walking program that includes interval workouts, and then graduate to a walk/jog program that safely gets you into the aerobic fitness zone. Sample programs are on page 58.

Swimming

Swimming is the fourth most popular sports activity in the U.S., and a good way to get regular aerobic activity, according to the Centers for Disease Control and Prevention (CDC). Here are some other CDC facts about swimming:

- Just two and a half hours per week can reduce the risk of chronic illness
- Swimmers have about half the risk of death compared to inactive people
- People report getting more enjoyment out of water-based exercise than exercising on land
- People can exercise longer in water than on land without increased effort or pain in joints or muscles

Drawbacks

Although an excellent method for becoming aerobically fit, swimming has its drawbacks. For most people, it takes time, effort, and possibly monetary expense to use a pool. And swimming laps, as opposed to other water-based activities, can be a solitary, even boring way to exercise for those not used to exercising or exercising alone. Finally, although swimming is an aerobic activity, it is not a weight-bearing exercise and doesn't promote bone health (it doesn't harm bone health—it just doesn't

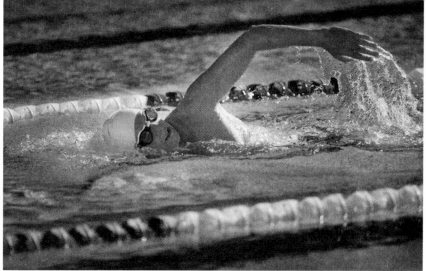

© Fuse | Thinkstock

Swimming is a popular low-impact, yet high-intensity, sports activity.

contribute to stronger bones).

Hot Spots and Remedies

The problem areas for swimmers are the shoulders and neck, in addition to fatigue and soreness. Avoid these potential injuries by mimicking the swimming motion with your arms as part of a dynamic warm up before getting into the water. Also include neck range-of-motion exercises.

Cycling

Riding a bicycle outside, or a stationary bike inside, qualifies on two counts: the aerobic challenge and ease of accessibility.

Cycling improves cardiovascular health as well as strength, balance, and flexibility.

© IPGGutenbergUKLtd | Thinkstock

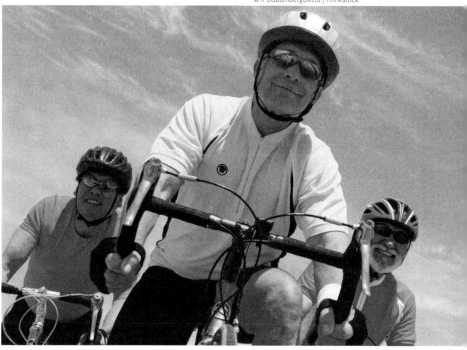

Cycling Safety

If you decide that cycling is going to be your activity, the National Institute on Aging offers the following safety guidelines:

- Visit a bike shop to get professionally fitted.
- While seated on the bike, your knee should be slightly bent when the pedal is in the lowest position.
- Check the brakes and tire pressure.
- Get a flashing red light for the rear of your bike, and lights or reflectors for the front.
- Wear bright clothing with reflective stripes and patches.
- Wear a helmet that fits.
- Avoid riding at night.
- Ride in the same direction as traffic.
- Stop at intersections, and signal when making turns.
- Watch for vehicles entering and leaving driveways.
- Yield to pedestrians, and alert them when close.

Adapted from Go4Life, National Institute on Aging at NIH

Benefits

Cycling is low impact, but is great for allowing you to control the frequency, intensity, and duration of your workouts. In addition to cardiovascular endurance, riding a bicycle also offers strength, flexibility, and balance training. Cycling does require some basic skills, including

Schwinn® Indoor Cycling Program

ZONE	% OF HR MAXIMUM	RATE OF PERCEIVED EXERTION
1	50–65	5–6 (easy/comfortable)
2	65–75	6–7 (challenging but comfortable)
3	75–85	7–8 (challenging and uncomfortable)
4	85–95	8–9 (breathless; not maximum, but winded)

knowing some basic safety guidelines (see "Cycling Safety").

Cycling programs for beginners and older adults are limited, but there are some you can follow for all-around aerobic fitness. For instance, the Schwinn® Indoor Cycling Program recommends a cardiovascular training program based on numbered intensity zones (see "Schwinn® Indoor Cycling Program"). Beginning and older exercisers should not get into zones 3 or 4 without consulting their doctor first. Many gyms also offer low-intensity spinning/indoor cycling classes for beginners and older adults.

Hot Spots and Remedies

Typical hot spots for cyclists are the neck, back, and wrists. Saddle soreness and overall muscle fatigue also are common. Dynamic warm ups and cool downs can help avoid problems and injuries to the quadriceps, hamstrings, calves, and abdominal muscles.

Water Aerobics

If you are comfortable in the water, but want a more varied exercise routine than swimming laps, water aerobics might be the right fit. This activity can build muscle tone, expend calories, and increase aerobic capacity. Water aerobics is particularly helpful for people with medical conditions like arthritis because exercises performed in water place less stress on the joints. Water provides resistance (and thus, strength training)

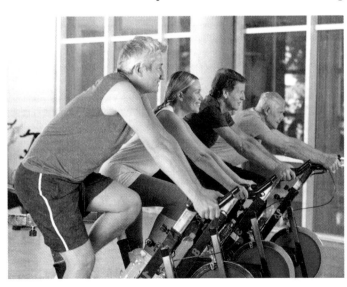

Spinning classes are great for seniors! They offer a low-impact workout that is consistent, stable, and safe.

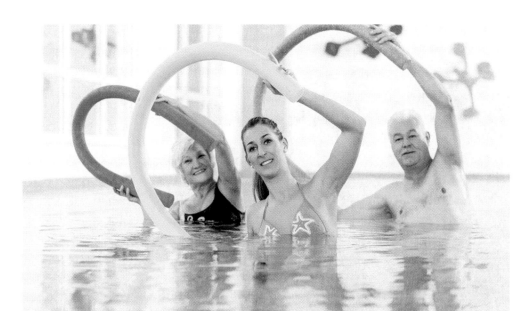

Water aerobics are ideal workouts for people with joint and mobility issues.

in every direction, and water exercises can be designed to fit individual needs.

Finally, you don't have to know how to swim to participate in a program, and most people do water aerobics in groups, so you get both physical and social benefits.

Variety Of Programs

The variety of exercises and programs is almost endless. For example, one Midwestern YMCA offers the following water-based choices:

- Aqua Arthritis
- Aquacise
- Aqua Pump
- Deep Water Aquacise
- Golden Aerobics
- Mobility in Motion
- Shallow Water Aerobics
- Water Strength and Endurance

What To Wear

Wear something that will streamline your movement in the pool. T-shirts and baggy pants cause too much drag. A one- or two-piece swimsuit works best. Your feet might need arch support, and some companies make aqua sneakers that have holes for water drainage. An old pair of gym shoes might offer the same support, but wash them before getting into the pool and use them only during water workouts.

A typical program moves the participant through a progressive sequence beginning with a warm up to a peak intensity period, and finishing with a cool-down session. Choose exercises you like, and add more later on for variety.

Water Exercise Options

Sample water aerobic exercise programs appear on page 59. For these workouts, move or push through the water, but only at a speed you can manage with control (without wavering or losing your stability).

Suggestions for repetitions and sets are for structure, safety, variety, and strength training, not necessarily aerobic fitness, which requires a heart rate in a target zone for an extended period of time. However, it's possible to improve strength, flexibility, balance, and cardiovascular fitness by doing the same exercises.

Hot Spots and Remedies

The whole body will be involved in water aerobics, so any area may have its share of normal muscle soreness. Warm up with calisthenics and out-of-water movements that you'll be doing

Many gyms host dance and aerobic classes designed for older adults.

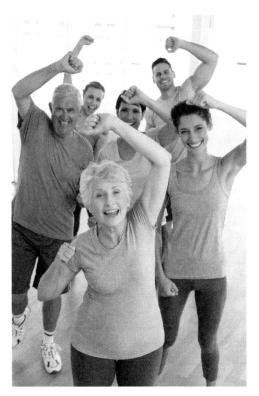

in the water. Take it slow. Begin with a few repetitions and one or two sets, then gradually work your way up to eight to 10 repetitions and two to three sets.

Dance Aerobics

More than 20 million Americans participate in aerobic exercise classes and many of them choose aerobic dancing. It is typically a one-hour workout that combines floor exercises and dance movements set to music. The hour should include a five- to 10-minute warm up and cool down.

One of the first and most popular dance programs was Jazzercise. It was introduced in the 1970s and is still out there in multiple platforms. According to its supporters, Jazzercise is "a fusion of jazz dance, aerobic exercise, resistance training, Pilates, yoga, and kickboxing."

There have been hundreds of variations since the aerobic dance explosion of the 1980s, but one that has been especially popular over the past decade is Zumba. It is, according to the Mayo Clinic, "a fitness program that combines Latin and international music with dance moves." Zumba routines incorporate

alternating fast and slow rhythms with resistance training. It would be classified as moderate aerobic activity for younger adults; moderate-to-vigorous for older exercisers.

A small study conducted at the University of Wisconsin-La Crosse and reported in the *Journal of Sports Science & Medicine* found that all participants in a Zumba experimental group reached ACSM aerobic exercise guidelines for percentage of heart rate maximum, with an average of 79 percent.

Pros and Cons

The advantages of dance aerobics are a solid, supervised aerobic workout, added enjoyment because of the music component, and exercising in the company of others if you join a group. Exercise is repetitious and can be boring, but that's not a problem in dance aerobics. The physical activity, group setting, and upbeat music tend to keep people engaged.

Perhaps the greatest advantage of dance aerobics is that you can participate in a class or group environment, or you can exercise at home, alone, and at your own pace with DVD programs.

The disadvantages, or perhaps obstacles, of group dance aerobics are identifying a program, being committed enough and able to get to a gym or fitness center on a regular basis, and doing the physical work required of aerobic dance. It is a challenging form of exercise, but all aerobic exercise should be challenging.

High-Impact, Low-Impact

Be sure to ask about the level of the group you are considering and whether the exercise is low-impact, high-impact, or high-low. Low-impact aerobics focus on a less demanding cardiovascular load over a longer period of time. One foot is always on the ground.

High-impact exercises get your heart rate closer to 80 to 85 percent of maximum level, but can involve stepping up on a platform, jumping, hopping, or other moves in which there is a greater impact on the bones and joints. Know that you don't have to jump in a class. You can simple walk or step the move for lower impact. Walking is low impact. Jogging, running, and in some cases, dance aerobics, are high-impact exercises.

High-low aerobic exercise combines both high and low impact moves, with the goal of getting you up, moving, and into the target heart rate zone.

If you are beginning a program, start with one that is low-impact, then decide if you want to stay at that level or move to a more aggressive routine. And remember, with dance aerobics, you do not have to do the movements perfectly. If you cannot keep up at first, it's okay to march or jog in place until you can pick up the next move.

Step Aerobics

Step aerobics is similar to dance aerobics, but requires you to step up and down on low platforms or boxes that range from four to 10 inches in height. The idea is to keep one foot on the ground, which is supposed to classify step aerobics as low-impact, but for some it may be a more challenging form of aerobics than dancing. Step aerobics falls somewhere between moderate to vigorous intensity.

A study published in the *Journal of Strength and Conditioning* examined the effects of a 12-week step aerobic training in a group of women with an average age of 63. The programs had a positive effect on waist circumference, upper and lower body strength, and cardiorespiratory fitness, among other measurements.

Hot Spots and Remedies

The higher the impact of aerobic exercises, the higher the injury rate. Among the most common injuries are plantar fasciitis, shin splints, stress fractures,

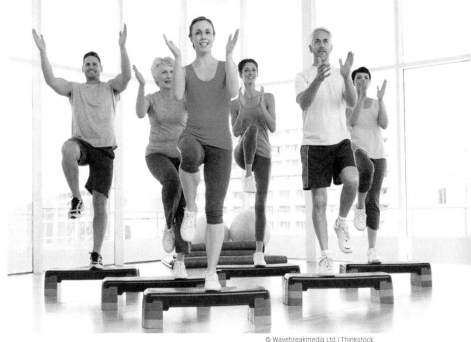

© Wavebreakmedia Ltd | Thinkstock

Step aerobics is a low-impact exercise that also builds lower body strength.

and Achilles tendon and calf pain. There is also a higher risk of falling with step aerobics.

Shoe selection, warming up, starting slowly and gradually increasing exercise intensity, frequency, and duration can reduce the risk. Adding strength, flexibility, and balance training to your comprehensive fitness program will further reduce the risk of all injuries even more.

Sports

Team and individual sports present a problem for middle-aged and older adults in terms of aerobic fitness. They either require too many people to play or, more importantly, don't provide enough continuous activity at an intensity level strenuous enough to get your heart into your target heart rate zone.

Some sports are relatively popular with older adults (golf and bowling, for example) and provide fitness benefits, such as flexibility, mobility, balance, and strength, but the cardiovascular component is simply not there (although golfers can get a better workout if they walk instead of riding in a cart).

Golfers can enjoy a good aerobic workout by walking and not riding in a cart.

© Studio Zanello/Ken Chernus Photography | Thinkstock

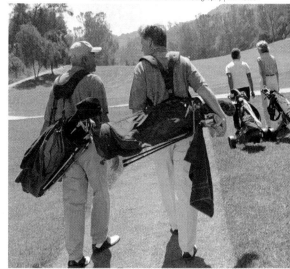

Tennis is one sport that can be aerobically beneficial, but there are restrictions. Even though singles is a stop-and-go game, it is considered an aerobic activity for most people. But it's also a high-impact activity, especially on hard courts, and some exercisers are better off doing low-impact aerobics for safety and injury prevention. Doubles in tennis provides a lower-impact workout, but in most cases does not reach the aerobic standard.

If you are a tennis player looking for a cardiovascular workout, consider a program called Cardio Tennis. It is a series of group lessons and activities that feature drills, a high-energy workout, player-friendly tennis balls, music, and heart rate monitors. Cardio Tennis is taught by a trained instructor, usually with a group of six to eight players, and includes a warm-up, aerobic exercise segments, and a cool down The emphasis is on aerobic activity more than tennis instruction, although you get some of both. Go to www.cardiotennis.com for more information.

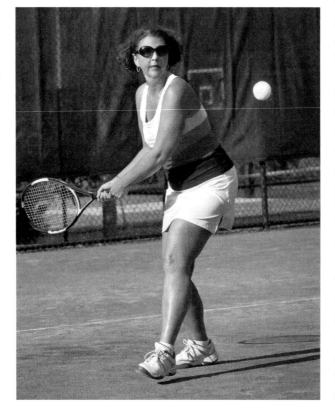

Cardio Tennis is a high-energy workout that emphasizes aerobic activity rather than tennis instruction.

Exercise Machines

Exercise machines mimic almost every sport and physical activity, and most can be incorporated into an aerobic exercise program. Depending on the machine, they can improve strength, power, flexibility, balance, and aerobic capacity.

All have disadvantages, however, including:

- Expense
- Repetitious nature of exercise machines that can lead to injuries,
- Boredom factor, which can result in some people using them less frequently or not using them at all
- Inaccurate feedback features

Any estimate of exercise intensity, calories burned, and other measurements depend on factors that machines cannot process (age, gender, health, and physical condition). You'll have to decide whether the advantages outweigh the disadvantages.

Elliptical Trainers

These are low-impact, safe for people with range-of-motion problems, and allow upper and lower body exercise simultaneously, but they are not weight-bearing and do not build strength.

Rowing Machines

These are particularly good for upper-body strength and flexibility. Although they involve low-impact exercise, they can easily get you into your target heart rate zone. However, they are not the best choice for people with back problems. Other "hot spots" are the knees and shoulders.

Treadmills

Treadmills are speed-adjustable for walkers, joggers, and runners. Other than changing speed and incline, treadmills don't offer much variety—there also is an increased fall risk when using a treadmill. Still, they are a staple exercise machine at most gyms and fitness centers and thus, easily accessible.

Recumbent Cycles

These are low-impact, take pressure off the back and legs, and give you support that other machines don't. They also leave your hands free, allowing you do other tasks. Unlike stationary bicycles, you cannot use your full body weight (or stand), so pushing the pedals can be harder. That's an advantage for some, a disadvantage for others.

Stationary Bicycles

Stationary bicycles are easy to use, convenient, not dependent on weather, and allow you to watch TV while exercising. They primarily exercise the legs and can get boring in a hurry. Stationary cycling at a moderate pace burns 450 to 500 calories per hour, depending on your weight.

Ergometers

Ergometers are used to strengthen and condition either the upper or lower body, and to get a cardiovascular workout by using only your arms or legs. They are used more in physical therapy settings, but can be found in many fitness facilities or gyms. They can be used to give your arms or legs a break, and for warming up. The machines can be an ideal choice for people with mobility issues or who are returning to exercise after an injury or long layoff.

Steppers

These are calorie-burners (as much as 600 per hour for a person who weighs 150 pounds). They are also an effective cardio exercise and are considered a more challenging workout than elliptical trainers. Steppers, however, involve impact and put a greater strain on knee joints than ellipticals.

Back To Basics

The average person is not going to do basic calisthenic-type exercises for 30 minutes or more at a time. But people who prefer to accumulate their 30 minutes or more of aerobic exercise per day in 10-minute bursts might consider combining some basic body-weight exercises. They include push-ups, step-ups, marching or jogging in place, jumping jacks, and lunges. None of them will work unless they get your heart rate into your target zone. Warm up for body-weight exercises as you would for any other aerobic activity.

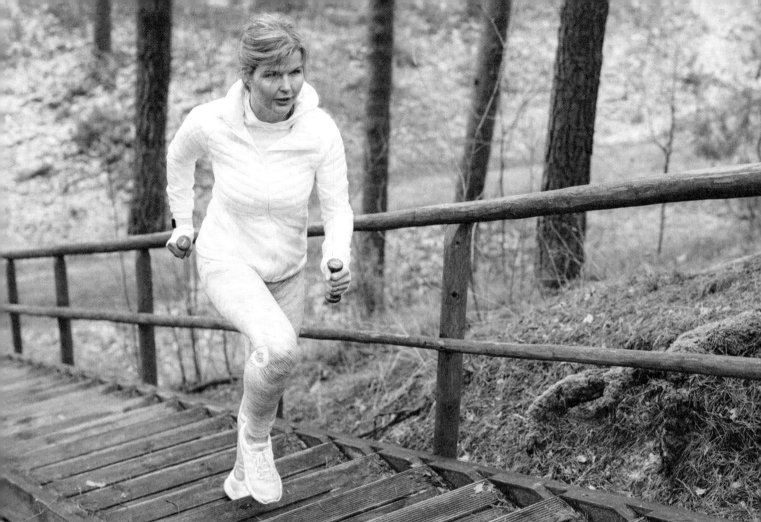

© Cecilie_Arcurs | Dreamstime

Climbing stairs and holding dumbbells (1-2 lbs.) are great ways to add resistance to your workout.

4 Minimize Injuries

The risk of injury as a result of aerobic exercise is small, but it's there. One of the few studies to address this issue found that among older adults, 14 percent reported injuries and 41 percent of the injuries were to lower extremities.

Among those who received instruction about how to avoid injuries, the injury rate was no higher for seniors than among middle-aged and younger adults (see "Exercise-Related Injury Rates Similar for Older, Middle-Aged, and Younger Adults").

Common lower body injuries, in addition to muscle strains, are shin splints, plantar fasciitis, blisters, sprains, knee pain, stress fractures, and muscle soreness, in no particular order.

Muscle Soreness

Some muscle soreness is to be expected when beginning an exercise program, but it should resolve itself within a couple of days. You can minimize it by warming up properly, gradually increasing exercise intensity and duration, and not overdoing it.

RESEARCH FINDING

Exercise-Related Injury Rates Similar for Older, Middle-Aged, and Younger Adults

Researchers at the University of Western Ontario studied a group of older men and women to determine the rate and types of exercise-related injuries they incurred. They found that 14 percent reported injuries, 41 percent of the injuries were to lower extremities, and that the most common injuries were overuse-related muscle strains. One-half of the injuries occurred during or after walking, possibly because walking was the most popular form of exercise. Seventy percent required medical attention, and 44 percent were not able to resume exercising immediately. The return-to-activity time varied from one to 182 days. The authors concluded that injury rates to older adults were about the same as in younger and middle-aged adults.

BMJ Open

Delayed onset muscle soreness (DOMS) is also a condition involving muscle overuse, and usually develops a day or two after an especially hard workout. While soreness after almost any vigorous exercise session is normal, DOMS is less common and probably indicates that you have stressed the muscle tissues beyond their normal capacity.

The discomfort begins at a muscle-tendon junction and spreads throughout the affected muscle. DOMS hurts for a couple of days, but it's not a serious condition and the symptoms will go away with rest.

Plantar Fasciitis

Plantar fasciitis is an inflammation of the fibrous tissue (called plantar fascia) that runs along the bottom surface of the foot from the heel to the base of the toes. "Heel spurs" or "stone bruises" may develop as a result of prolonged inflammation. No one knows for sure how or why it develops, but plantar fasciitis affects women more often than men, as well as people who are overweight, have flat feet, or work in a job that requires walking or standing on a hard

Plantar Fasciitis

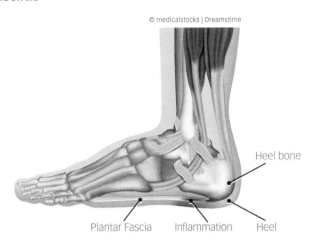

© medicalstocks | Dreamstime

Heel bone

Plantar Fascia   Inflammation   Heel

surface. Other contributing factors may include excessive foot pronation (ankle rolling inward), wearing shoes that are worn down at the heel, and running on uphill surfaces. The injury may involve a cumulative overload on the feet that causes microtears and degeneration of the plantar fascia tissue.

The first line of treatment is a home-based program of stretching the plantar fascia and the Achilles tendon three times a day. Two effective stretches are the plantar fascia stretch, and the tennis ball massage.

PLANTAR FASCIA STRETCH

- Sit down, cross the affected leg/foot across the other, just above the knee.
- Grasp the toes/top of the affected foot and pull back toward the body.
- Hold for 10-30 seconds, three repetitions.

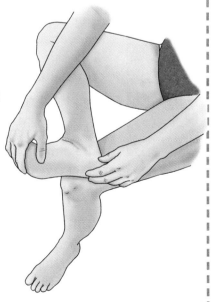

Illustrations by Alayna Paquette

TENNIS BALL MASSAGE

- In a seated position, place a tennis ball or large dowel under the foot.
- Roll the ball forward and backward, stretching the undersurface of the foot.
- Avoid excessive downward pressure.

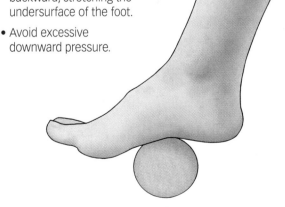

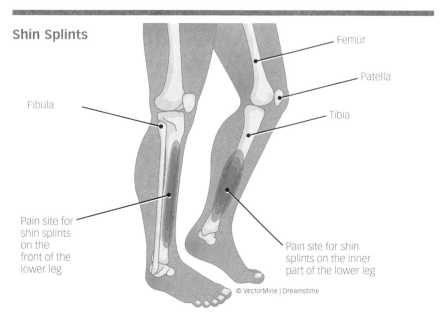

Shin Splints

Femur

Patella

Tibia

Fibula

Pain site for shin splints on the front of the lower leg

Pain site for shin splints on the inner part of the lower leg

© VectorMine | Dreamstime

Shin Splints

Medial tibial stress syndrome, also called tibial pain syndrome but more commonly called shin splints, is a term for pain in the front or inner part of the lower leg. Shin splints are one of the most common sports and exercise injuries, and can develop in everyone from elite long-distance runners to recreational athletes and regular exercisers.

Shin splints can involve inflamed muscles, tendons, and the thin layer of tissue that covers the bone. Although they can be painful enough to take you out of action for a while, most cases of shin splints can be treated with conservative treatment, such as applying ice packs to the area four to six times a day for 10 minutes at a time, rest, and over-the-counter pain relief and anti-inflammatory medications.

You might be able to avoid shin splints by walking or running on a slightly cushioned surface, such as a running track or grass. Asphalt is better than concrete. Minimize the risk by wearing athletic shoes that provide support through the sole of the foot and the arch and possibly by using shoe orthotics (inserts). Changing shoes every four to six months might also help, as will the Calf Stretch (see Exercise 6, page 53).

Blisters

The most likely places for blisters to develop on aerobic exercisers are on the feet. Shoes that don't fit properly, differences in surfaces, heat, dampness, friction, and increased frequency of activity could all lead to blisters.

Most blisters heal by themselves when the source of friction is removed. If the top area of the skin remains intact, a doughnut-like pad placed over the top protects the skin and relieves the discomfort.

If the skin has already been removed, treat the area as an abrasion. Wash it with mild soapy water or an antiseptic, then cover it with a bandage. Ask about over-the-counter medicated blister dressings at a pharmacy. If a blister or other sore does not heal on its own, see a physician.

Strained (Pulled) Quadriceps

The quadriceps are a group of four muscles (thigh muscles) in front of the upper leg that work together with the hamstrings (behind the upper leg) to

If you suffer from pain in your shin when you exercise, you may have shin splints. See your doctor before continuing your workout routine or try something less taxing on the shins.

© Dirima | Thinkstock

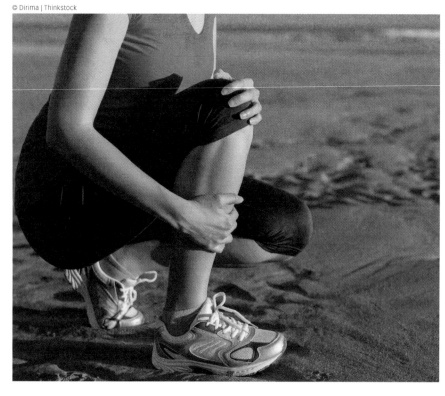

extend and bend the leg. Strong quadriceps are important for walkers, joggers, runners, swimmers, and other exercisers.

Injuries to the quads are among the most common (and treatable) in exercisers at all levels. A strained quadriceps muscle involves a partial or complete tear of one of those four muscles, or their tendons, when stretched beyond their normal limits. Muscle strains, including those involving the quadriceps, are graded one, two, or three by physicians, according to the severity of the injury.

The injury often happens when a person needs to accelerate. The quads are placed under more force than they can withstand at the moment, and the muscle fibers, tendons, or both begin to tear away from the bone where they are attached.

When the muscles are fatigued, overused, or not adequately warmed up, they are at increased risk of a strain. An imbalance between weak quadriceps and stronger hamstrings (a condition that is common among runners) can also cause the injury, as can simply having tight quadriceps.

The initial treatment is rest, and cold packs for 15 to 20 minutes, three to four times a day for the first 48 to 72 hours. After that, moist heat for the next 48- to 72-hour period, three to four times a day, followed by gentle stretching of the quadricep muscles. Use pillows to elevate the affected leg during the first day and night.

Aspirin, acetaminophen, ibuprofen, and naproxen may relieve pain. All but acetaminophen reduce inflammation.

Strained (Pulled) Hamstring

The hamstring muscles are the three muscles that run down the back of the thigh. They attach to the lower pelvis and to the back of the leg just below the knee. Those three muscles, working

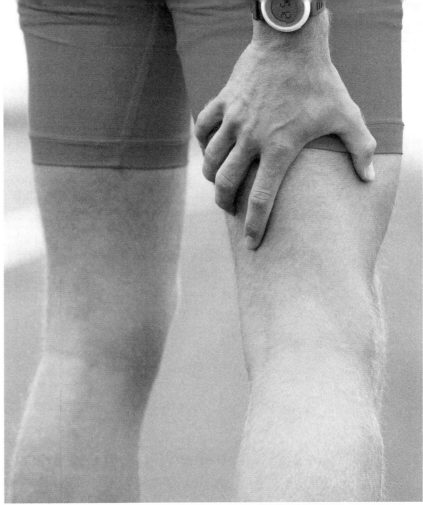

© Martinmark | Dreamstime

You may be able to prevent a strained hamstring with proper warm-up and cool-down exercises.

in concert with the quadriceps on the front of the legs, allow your legs to straighten out at the hip joint and bend at the knees.

Both the quadriceps and hamstrings are active throughout most of the aerobic activity described above. During different phases of movement, one muscle group may be more active than the other, and when knee stability is required they may be contracting simultaneously. A cold (not properly warmed up) muscle that is required to contract at maximum intensity is at high risk for injury.

You'll know if you've pulled a hamstring by the severe pain behind the upper leg or buttock, possible muscle spasms, bruising and tenderness, and swelling. With a complete tear, you may feel a knot of muscle on the back of your leg.

A strained hamstring can be painful and hard to heal, but in many cases are preventable. The injury is a strain or tear in the muscles and tendons that run along the back part of the upper legs. Rest, ice applications, elevation, and compression wraps are first aid treatments. Aspirin, acetaminophen, ibuprofen, and naproxen may relieve the pain. To reduce the risk of a pulled hamstring:

- Do not increase exercise intensity, frequency, or duration more than 10 percent in one week
- Be sure to stretch the hamstrings adequately after exercise (see Hamstring Stretch, Exercise 2, page 52)
- Stop exercising if you feel tightness in the back of your legs
- Allow extra warm-up time in cold weather

Strained (Pulled) Calf Muscle

The two large muscles in the back of the lower leg (soleus and gastrocnemius) are called calf muscles, and they are at risk every time an exerciser pushes off—even if the activity is just walking. When the muscles are stretched beyond their normal capacity, the muscle fibers tear away from the tendon. Joggers, runners, and tennis players are particularly susceptible, but any exerciser who "pushes off" can suffer the injury.

The symptoms are sudden pain in the back of the lower leg between the knee and heel, pain when pushing off, stiffness, weakness, and bruising. As with other strains, rest, ice, compression, elevation, and over-the-counter pain medications are the initial treatments.

Stress Fractures

Among the people who are at higher risk for stress fractures—small cracks in a bone—are sedentary individuals who begin a demanding exercise program, people who have diabetes or rheumatoid arthritis, and those who have osteoporosis or other conditions that result in weakened bones or decreased bone density.

While a stress fracture is typically an overuse injury, it could happen with nothing more than a change of activity.

A doctor may make a stress fracture diagnosis with an x-ray or CT scan, but the symptoms are a dull ache following exercise, swelling, pain that decreases only with rest and increases with activity, pain that gets progressively worse, and an area that is painful when pressure is applied.

The first treatment is stopping the activity that caused the injury, and not resuming for as long as six to eight weeks. Most stress fractures heal with time, and orthopedic supports like shoe inserts, or boot walkers, depending on the location of the injury.

Sprained Ankle

The ankle is the most frequently injured part of the body among exercisers. The severity of the injury ranges from one that allows the person to return to normal activity in a few days to an injury that keeps a person out of action for weeks at a time. Those who have had a sprained ankle are the ones most likely to suffer the same injury again.

A sprained ankle is a stretch, tear, or rupture of at least one of the ligaments that hold the bones of the ankle joint together. The tears may be microscopic or so large that they represent a complete disruption of the fibers. One of the ligaments that wraps around the

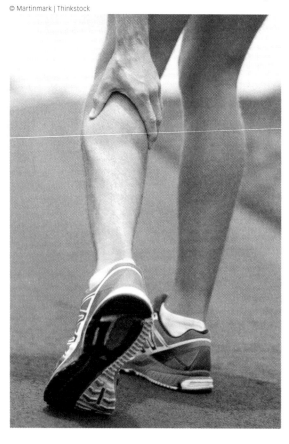

If you feel sudden pain in the back of your lower leg, you may have a strained or pulled calf muscle.

© Martinmark | Thinkstock

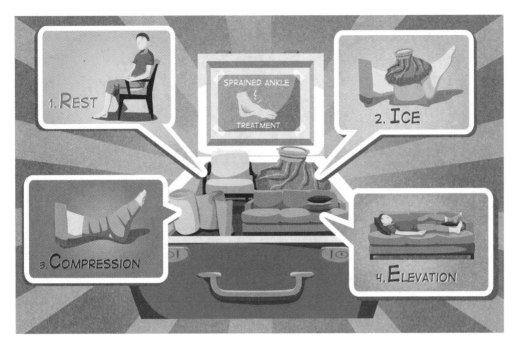

The remedy for a sprained ankle is RICE: rest, ice, compression, and elevation.

outside of the ankle is the weakest of the ankle ligaments and is the one most frequently injured. It is possible that all three ligaments supporting the ankle, from front to back, may be sprained.

Symptoms vary according to the severity and grade (one, two, or three) of the sprain. The best-case scenario is mild pain, localized swelling, and tenderness, but no instability. You can walk, but don't try to jog or jump. Grade two and three sprains involve greater pain, a popping sound, bleeding, bruising, ankle instability, and difficulty in walking.

First aid is rest, ice, compression with an elastic bandage, wrap, or support device, elevation, and pain medication.

Protective measures include wearing protective shoes with side-to-side support, bracing or taping the ankle, and following the 10 percent rule (see page 25).

Cramps

Nine out of 10 cramps involve the quadriceps, hamstrings, and calves. The symptoms are unmistakable: sudden, involuntary, and painful muscle contractions. They can be caused by fatigue, hot and humid weather, prolonged overuse, dehydration, and electrolyte deficiencies. Electrolytes are potassium, calcium, and sodium, and people who take diuretics (used to treat hypertension) may develop an electrolyte imbalance.

Methods of relieving cramps include stretching the affected muscle group, applying pressure, and/or massaging it. A common mistake is trying to resume exercise immediately after the pain subsides. It won't work, and the muscle is likely to cramp again. If cramps persist, apply cold packs for 15 to 20 minutes, three to four times a day. (See "What To Do About Muscle Cramps.")

What To Do About Muscle Cramps

- Stop the activity that triggered the cramp.
- Gently stretch the muscle that is cramping.
- Massage the cramping muscle.
- Apply heat to tense or tight muscles.
- Apply cold applications to sore or tender muscles.
- Drink plenty of fluids before, during, and after vigorous exercise.

Adapted from the American Academy of Orthopaedic Surgeons

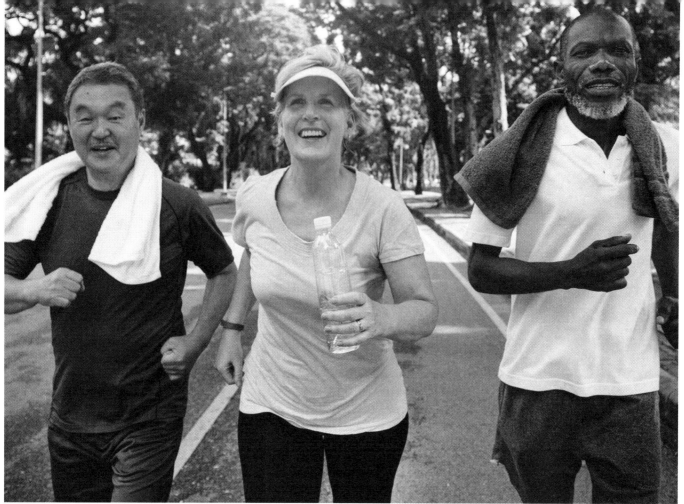
© Rawpixelimages | Thinkstock

Always start with five to 10 minutes of warm-up before attempting any exercise routine.

Avoid Ballistic Stretching

Unless you are an elite athlete, the one kind of stretching to avoid is called ballistic. Ballistic stretches involve rapid, bouncing movement that moves the joint beyond its normal range of motion or a range of motion limited by muscle tightness. Ballistic stretching can cause injury and soreness, and it doesn't allow enough time for the muscles tissues to adapt to the stretch. Instead of relaxing the muscle, it increases tension and makes it hard to stretch the surrounding connective tissues. The takeaway messages: no ballistic stretching, and no bouncing.

Warm Up

Regardless of the activity, every workout should begin with a dynamic warm up. The more prepared the body is, the less likely it is to get injured.

Devote about five to 10 minutes to a proper dynamic warm up. The actual warm up varies from person to person, but the goal is the same: break a sweat, gradually elevate the heart rate, and increase circulation.

Light calisthenics, slow-paced swimming or cycling, moderately-paced walking, and jogging can be effective warm ups. Another method is to move the body through a range of motion that mimics the exercise you will be doing.

Golfers and tennis players had this stage figured out a long time ago. What better way to warm the muscles up for golf than by first going through the motions on a driving range or hitting groundstrokes, volleys, lobs, smashes, and serves before a tennis match?

But do not confuse warming up with stretching, especially ballistic stretching (see "Avoid Ballistic Stretching"). You never want to stretch muscles when they are cold. Instead, save proper stretching for *after* your aerobic workout to reduce soreness, increase recovery time, and lower your risk of injury. There is also evidence that this kind of proper stretching increases range of motion.

Cool Down

Following an aerobic workout, don't just stop. Take a few minutes to cool down. It helps prevent blood pooling in your legs, avoids the risk of a sudden drop in blood pressure, and allows your heart rate to begin returning to normal in a controlled manner.

One suggestion is to cool down until your pulse rate drops below 120 beats per minute. Your level of fitness is improving if your recovery time is declining.

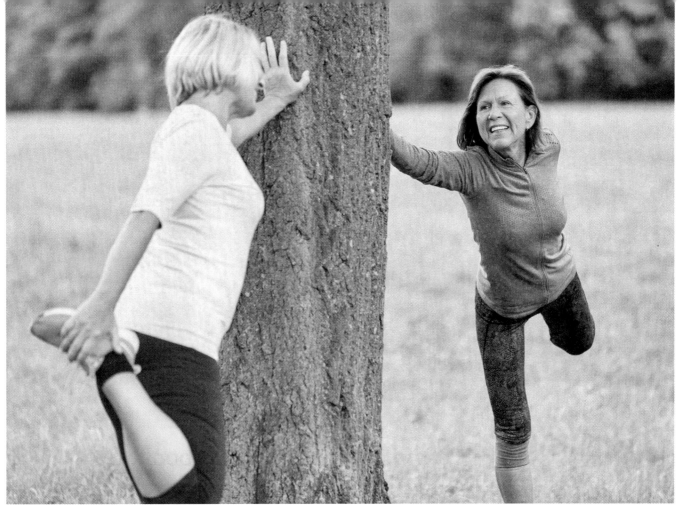

Walk, Run, Swim, Cycle

Walk slowly for five to 10 minutes after an aerobic walk. Cool down with a five- to 10-minute brisk walk/normal-paced walk after running. Swim laps for five to 10 minutes at a slower pace. Ride your bike around the block at a leisurely pace.

Just as you gradually warm up before an aerobic activity, you should gradually cool down afterward. Put a warm-up jacket on for a few minutes, even if the weather is hot. Avoid abrupt changes in body temperature.

Static Stretching

Finally, end your cool down by devoting several minutes to static stretching. Static stretches involve gently stretching a muscle or muscle group to a point of resistance and holding (not bouncing) the position for at least five to 10 seconds. UCLA physical therapists recommend it for muscles known to be at risk of injury in a particular activity, for muscles that have been previously injured, and for preventing diminished flexibility.

For aerobic activity, the muscles and muscle groups you should focus on include core/abdominals, quadriceps, hamstrings, and calves (see "Post-Exercise Static Stretching Routine").

Take A Break

Listen to your body, says the American College of Sports Medicine. Pain is a signal that something is not right. Take a break. Cross-train with a different activity. Exercise at a much lower intensity. Adding variety to your exercise schedule prevents overuse for some muscles and challenges others.

After completing your physical activity, cool down and stretch your muscles.

Post-Exercise Static Stretching Routine

Static stretching helps to avoid muscle soreness, improve recovery time, and reduce the risk of strains or injury. The following four exercises on pages XX and XX target the main muscles of aerobic activity. Do them after every aerobic workout:

- **Exercise 1:** Lunges
- **Exercise 2:** Hamstring Stretches
- **Exercise 3:** Sitting Twists
- **Exercise 6:** Calf Stretch

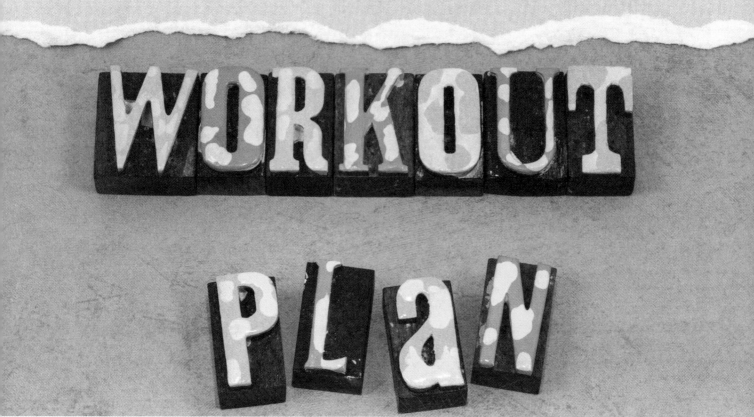

Now that you know what to do, it's time to put your plan into action!

5 Easy Exercises & Workbook

This chapter outlines everything you need to begin an aerobic fitness routine. It includes programs for three areas of aerobics: walk/jog, water aerobics, and gym/sports aerobic activities.

Programs
Walk/Jog
There are three programs from which to choose.
- **Walking Program 1** is for people who are not quite active, returning to exercise after a long layoff, or have some mobility issues.
- **Walking Program 2** includes periods where you increase your walking to a brisk pace followed by slow walking or rest. This is best for those who already have some foundation of fitness or are ready to move up from Walking Program 1.
- **Walk/Jog Program 3** is similar to Program 2, but includes jogging. This is for those who are ready to move up from Program 2 or are already conditioned to begin a more robust aerobic routine.

Water Aerobics
If you have access to a pool and are interested in a different type of aerobic workout, these four programs may be for you.

Gym/Sport Aerobic Activities
Gyms offer a variety of aerobic machines you can use for 30-minute workouts. Most also host classes, some of which may be designed for seniors. Many sports can be aerobic too, like swimming, tennis, and cycling.

Cross-Training
Cross-training is essential for safe and effective aerobic fitness, so we have created an eight-exercise workout for alternating days. They help reduce soreness and lower your risk of injury.

Two-Week Workbook
For the sample two-week workbook, we have filled out routines that cover each of these areas. These are only suggestions and you can mix and match or even repeat as you like.

CROSS-TRAINING EXERCISES

WATER AEROBIC EXERCISES

Exercise illustrations on pages 52–57 by Alayna Paquette

LUNGES

EXERCISE 1

- Stand with feet hip-width apart and take one long step forward, about 12-18 inches.

- Bend the front knee, dropping the back knee as close to the floor as possible. Do not allow the front knee to extend past the toes.

- Hold for 10 to 30 seconds. Slowly return to the starting position, relax, and repeat the movement eight to 10 times.

- Two to three sets for each leg.

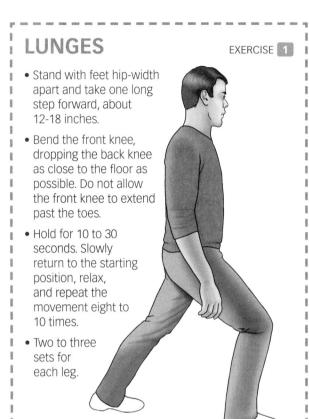

COOL-DOWN STATIC STRETCH

HAMSTRING STRETCH

EXERCISE 2

- Sit on the ground with legs extended in front.

- Lean forward and extend both arms and hands toward your toes. Keep your back flat and not rounded.

- Hold for five to 10 seconds, relax, and return to the starting position.

- Repeat two to three times.

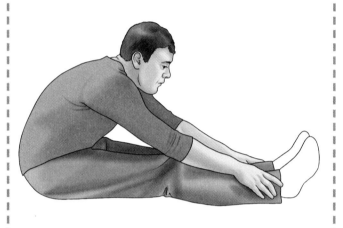

COOL-DOWN STATIC STRETCH

SITTING TWIST

EXERCISE 3

- Stand or sit erect in a straight-back chair.

- Cross your arms and rotate your shoulders to one side as far as possible without discomfort.

- Hold for one second, return to the starting position, and repeat eight to 12 times.

- Repeat the movement on the other side.

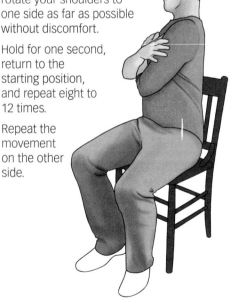

COOL-DOWN STATIC STRETCH

MODIFIED PUSH-UPS

EXERCISE 4

- Lie on your stomach, palms on the floor at about shoulder width.

- Slowly raise your upper body until your arms are fully extended, with back straight. If this is too challenging at first, you may bend your knees and lift the upper two-thirds of your body.

- Begin with four to five repetitions and work up to eight to 10 repetitions; complete two to three sets.

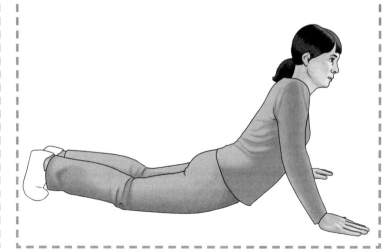

HEEL RAISES

- Hold a three- to eight-pound dumbbell in each hand, arms down, palms in.
- Stand with your toes on a secure surface.
- Rise slowly on your toes while keeping your body erect and knees straight.
- Return to the starting position and repeat the movement eight to 10 times.

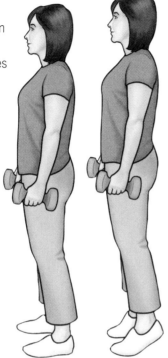

CALF STRETCH

- Place your left foot forward and the other foot back, arms extended, and hands against a wall.
- Bend your left knee while keeping the back heel in contact with the floor. Hold five to 10 seconds, and return to the starting position.
- Eight to 10 repetitions for each leg; two to three sets.

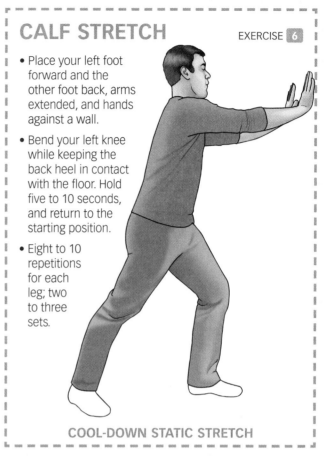

COOL-DOWN STATIC STRETCH

OVERHEAD REACH

- Interlock your fingers.
- Lift your arms overhead and rotate your wrists so the palms are facing up.
- Extend your arms as far upward as possible without straining and hold for 20 to 30 seconds.
- Repeat two to three times.

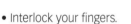

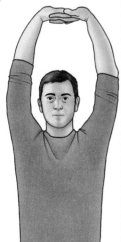

BACK EXTENSIONS

- Begin from an all-fours position on the floor.
- Slowly lift your left arm and right leg, hold for five seconds, then return to the starting position.
- Now slowly lift your right arm and left leg, hold for five seconds, then return to the starting position to complete one rep.
- Repeat eight to 10 times, rest, and complete a second set of eight to 10.

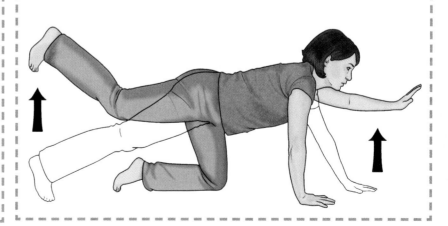

SIDE STEPS

EXERCISE 9

- Feet together, arms at your sides in waist-high or shoulder-deep water.

- Brace your spine and take a big step to the side with your right leg.

- At the same time, move your hands upward and out to your sides.

- Bring your left leg to meet your right leg with hands moving back to your sides.

- Repeat the sequence and move across the length of the pool.

- Repeat the same exercise, starting with the left leg to cross the pool in the opposite direction.

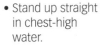

LEG PENDULUM

EXERCISE 10

- Back against the wall of the pool, arms on edge for support.

- Legs together, forward, and in front, head and eyes straight ahead.

- Swing both legs as far to the right as possible, then to your left.

- Complete four to five repetitions and two to three sets.

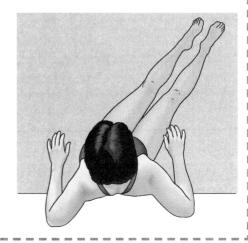

WATER MARCHING

EXERCISE 11

- Stand up straight in chest-high water.

- Make continuous strides, as if marching in place.

- Extend your arms as much as possible with each step.

- Complete a two-minute march, rest one minute, and repeat two to three times.

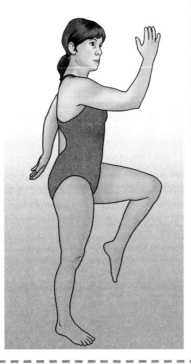

WATER LUNGES

EXERCISE 12

- Stand parallel to the wall of the pool, left arm on the edge for support.

- Lunge forward with your left leg while slightly lifting the heel of your back leg off the bottom of the pool. Do not extend your front knee past your toes.

- Return to the starting position and complete eight to 10 repetitions.

- Change positions and complete eight to 10 repetitions with the opposite leg for one set.

- Work up to two to three sets.

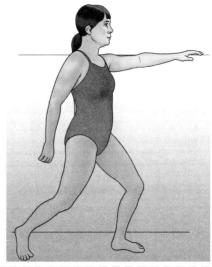

SHOULDER CLAP

- Standing in water just over shoulder height, extend your arms to the sides as far as possible.
- Bring your arms and hands forward just under the surface of the water, as though pushing them together to clap your hands.
- When your hands touch, force them back to the starting position.
- Repeat 10 to 20 times.

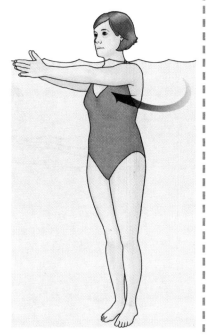

JUMPING JACKS

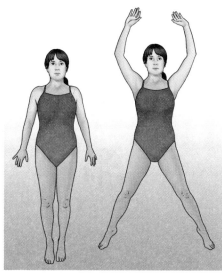

- With feet together and arms at your side, jump and push both feet out to the sides into a wide stride position.
- At the same time, lift your arms out of the water and overhead.
- Jump again and return to the starting position.
- Complete four to five repetitions to make one set, and do two to three sets.

KARATE PUNCH

- Shoulder-high water, elbows in, flexed at 90 degrees, fists clenched at sides.
- Punch the right arm 10 to 20 times, forcefully until it is fully extended. Repeat the punch 10 to 20 times.
- Stop, rest, and punch in the same motion with the left arm 10 to 20 times.
- Do one to three sets.

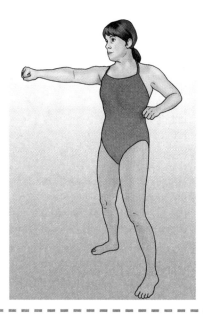

FRONT KICKS

- With feet shoulder-width apart, lift the right leg (flexing the hip) as high as possible without straining and while keeping a good posture.
- Return to the starting position.
- Repeat the movement with the left leg to complete one repetition. Do four to five reps to finish one set.
- Rest then complete two to three sets.

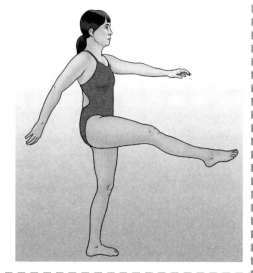

CORNER KICKS

EXERCISE **17**

- With feet shoulder-width apart, lift the left leg and then rotate it toward the diagonal corner of the pool at a 45-degree angle. Return to starting position.
- Lift the right leg and repeat the movement to the other diagonal corner to complete one repetition.
- Do four to five repetitions for one set. Rest then complete two to three sets.

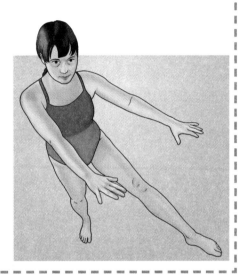

MINI SQUATS

EXERCISE **18**

- Stand in waist-deep water, supported by a bar or edge of the pool, if necessary.
- Sit back as if sitting in a chair (but only a quarter of the way down), making sure your knees do not come too forward past your toes.
- Use your legs (not your arms) to rise out of the squat.
- Work up to eight to 10 repetitions and do two to three sets.

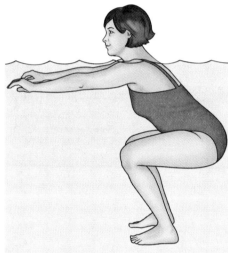

SCISSOR KICKS

EXERCISE **19**

- Stand with legs out in chest-high water, back to the side of the pool, arms on poolside for support.
- Use a scissor motion to alternately cross one leg in front of the other.
- Do four to five repetitions for one set. Complete two to three sets.

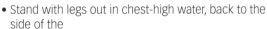

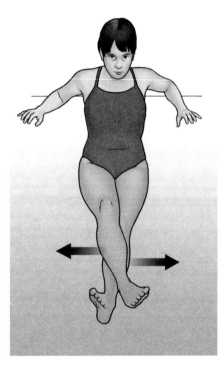

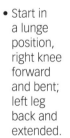

FLY-BACKS

EXERCISE **20**

- Start in a lunge position, right knee forward and bent; left leg back and extended.
- Arms forward at chest height, palms touching.
- Open your arms straight out and to the sides. Return to the starting position to complete one repetition.
- Do four to five repetitions to complete one set. Rest, then do two to three sets.

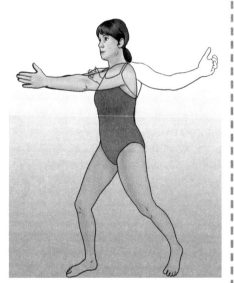

HAMSTRING CURLS EXERCISE 21

- Stand within arms length of the poolside for support, if needed.
- Extend your arms out to the side.
- Keeping knees together, bend your right knee and curl your lower leg up toward the buttocks.
- Return to starting position and repeat four to five times.
- Switch legs and repeat to complete one set.
- Do two to three sets.

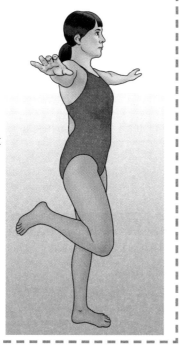

KICKBACKS EXERCISE 22

- Stand at arms length away from the side of the pool.
- Lean forward and place both hands on the poolside.
- Raise your right leg and swing it back, knees slightly bent. Return to the starting position.
- Repeat four to five times, then switch legs to complete one set.
- Do two to three sets.

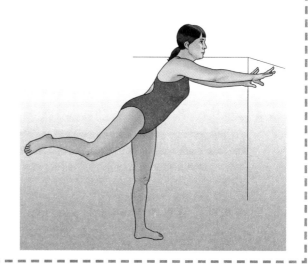

CROSS-COUNTRY SKI EXERCISE 23

- Stand in waist-to-chest-deep water, right foot forward, left foot back.
- Left arm reaching forward but under the water, right arm reaching back.
- Brace your spine, hop up, and bring your left leg forward while pressing the right leg back in a cross-country skiing motion.
- Scoop and press your palms forward and back with each stride.
- Repeat four to five times for one set.
- Do two to three sets.

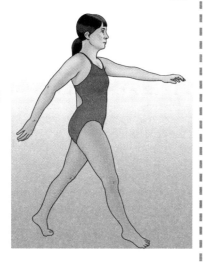

KNEE LIFTS EXERCISE 24

- Place your feet shoulder width apart.
- Lift the right leg up to approximately 90 degrees by flexing at the hip, left knee slightly bent. Raise your left arm for support.
- Repeat with the left leg and right arm.
- Do four to five repetitions, rest, and complete two to three sets.

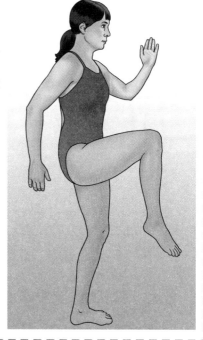

WATER AEROBICS

EASY EXERCISES

Sample Walking Program 1

This is only a guide. Your walking sessions may be longer or shorter based on your ability and the advice of your doctor. If you are walking fewer than three times per week, give yourself more than two weeks before adding more.

WEEKS	WARM-UP TIME Walk slowly	BRISK-WALK TIME	COOL-DOWN TIME Walk slowly	TOTAL TIME
1–2	5 minutes	5 minutes	5 minutes	15 minutes
3–4	5 minutes	10 minutes	5 minutes	20 minutes
5–6	5 minutes	15 minutes	5 minutes	25 minutes
7–8	5 minutes	20 minutes	5 minutes	30 minutes
9–10	5 minutes	25 minutes	5 minutes	35 minutes

Source: Weight-control Information Network from the National Institute of Diabetes and Digestive and Kidney Diseases

Sample Walking Program 2

During each session, try not to stop before the end of the total time goal.

WEEKS	WARM-UP TIME Slow, moderate pace	BRISK-ACTIVITY TIME			COOL-DOWN TIME Slow, moderate pace	TOTAL TIME
		Walk at brisk pace	Walk slowly or rest	Walk at brisk pace		
1–2	5 min.	5 min. or less	3 min.	5 min.	5 min.	23 min.
3–4	5 min.	8-10 min.	3 min.	8-10 min.	5 min.	29-33 min.
5–6	5 min.	10-15 min.	3 min.	10-15 min.	5 min.	33-43 min.

Source: National Heart, Lung, and Blood Institute

Sample Walk/Jog Program 3

During each session, try not to stop before the end of the total time goal.

WEEK	WARM-UP TIME Walk slowly or do a dynamic warm up	BRISK-ACTIVITY TIME				COOL-DOWN TIME Walk slowly	TOTAL TIME
		Walk briskly	Jog	Walk briskly	Jog		
1	5 min.	10 min.				5 min.	20 min.
2	5 min.	5 min.	1 min.	5 min.	1 min.	5 min.	22 min.
3	5 min.	5 min.	3 min.	5 min.	3 min.	5 min.	26 min.
4	5 min.	4 min.	5 min.	4 min.	5 min.	5 min.	28 min.
5	5 min.	4 min.	5 min.	4 min.	5 min.	5 min.	28 min.
6	5 min.	4 min.	6 min.	4 min.	6 min.	5 min.	30 min.
7	5 min.	4 min.	7 min.	4 min.	7 min.	5 min.	32 min.
8	5 min.	4 min.	8 min.	4 min.	8 min.	5 min.	34 min.
9	5 min.	4 min.	9 min.	4 min.	9 min.	5 min.	36 min.

Source: National Heart, Lung, and Blood Institute

EASY EXERCISES

Sample Water Aerobics Programs

It's fine to switch out exercises if you like some more than others. However, the advantage of repeating exercises is to measure your progress. Note that the total time for each exercise is an estimate. You may need more or less time at first depending on your conditioning.

Sample Water Aerobics Program 1

ACTIVITY	APPROX. TIME
Warm up (jogging, calisthenics, dynamic swimming-related movement)	5-10 minutes
Exercise 11 Water marching	10 minutes
Exercise 9 Side steps	5 minutes
Exercise 15 Karate punch	5 minutes
Exercise 21 Hamstring curls	5 minutes
Exercise 14 Jumping jacks	5 minutes
Cool down (walking, static stretches, slow-pace lap swimming)	5-10 minutes

Sample Water Aerobics Program 2

ACTIVITY	APPROX. TIME
Warm up (jogging, calisthenics, dynamic swimming-related movement)	5-10 minutes
Exercise 11 Water marching	5-7 minutes
Exercise 9 Side steps	5-7 minutes
Exercise 16 Front kicks	2-3 minutes
Exercise 20 Fly-backs	5 minutes
Exercise 15 Karate punch	5 minutes
Cool down (walking, static stretches, slow-pace lap swimming)	5-10 minutes

Sample Water Aerobics Program 3

ACTIVITY	APPROX. TIME
Warm up (jogging, calisthenics, dynamic swimming-related movement)	5-10 minutes
Exercise 24 Knee lifts	5-7 minutes
Exercise 18 Mini squats	5-7 minutes
Exercise 17 Corner kicks	2-3 minutes
Exercise 19 Scissor kicks	5 minutes
Exercise 23 Cross-country ski	5 minutes
Cool down (walking, static stretches, slow-pace lap swimming)	5-10 minutes

Sample Water Aerobics Program 4

ACTIVITY	APPROX. TIME
Warm up (jogging, calisthenics, dynamic swimming-related movement)	5-10 minutes
Exercise 10 Leg pendulum	5-7 minutes
Exercise 12 Water lunges	5-7 minutes
Exercise 13 Shoulder clap	2-3 minutes
Exercise 22 Kickbacks	5 minutes
Exercise 23 Cross-country ski	5 minutes
Cool down (walking, static stretches, slow-pace lap swimming)	5-10 minutes

WEEK #1

EXERCISE DAY OF THE WEEK	GYM/SPORT ACTIVITY (SEE PAGES 31–41)	WALK AND WALK/JOG (SEE PAGE 58)	WATER AEROBICS (SEE PAGE 59)	☑ CHECK WHEN COMPLETED	COMMENTS
MONDAY		✔*			*Choose either program one, two, or three depending on your current fitness level.
TUESDAY (CROSS-TRAINING)					Complete the eight-exercise routine on pages 52 and 53.
WEDNESDAY	✔*				*Choose a gym aerobic machine, dance class, or sport activity. Do 30 minutes.
THURSDAY (CROSS-TRAINING)					Complete the eight-exercise routine on pages 52 and 53.
FRIDAY			✔*		*Choose one of the four water aerobic programs.
SATURDAY		REST			
SUNDAY		REST			

WEEK #2

EXERCISE DAY OF THE WEEK	GYM/SPORT ACTIVITY (SEE PAGES 31–41)	WALK AND WALK/JOG (SEE PAGE 58)	WATER AEROBICS (SEE PAGE 59)	☑ CHECK WHEN COMPLETED	COMMENTS
MONDAY	✔*				*Choose a gym aerobic machine, dance class, or sport activity. Do 30 minutes.
TUESDAY (CROSS-TRAINING)					Complete the eight-exercise routine on pages 52 and 53.
WEDNESDAY			✔*		*Choose one of the four water aerobic programs.
THURSDAY (CROSS-TRAINING)					Complete the eight-exercise routine on pages 52 and 53.
FRIDAY		✔*			*Choose either program one, two, or three depending on your current fitness level.
SATURDAY		REST			
SUNDAY		REST			

EXERCISE DAY OF THE WEEK	GYM/SPORT ACTIVITY (SEE PAGES 31–41)	WALK AND WALK/JOG (SEE PAGE 58)	WATER AEROBICS (SEE PAGE 59)	☑ CHECK WHEN COMPLETED	COMMENTS
MONDAY		✓*			*Choose either program one, two, or three depending on your current fitness level.
TUESDAY (CROSS-TRAINING)					Complete the eight-exercise routine on pages 52 and 53.
WEDNESDAY	✓*				*Choose a gym aerobic machine, dance class, or sport activity. Do 30 minutes.
THURSDAY (CROSS-TRAINING)					Complete the eight-exercise routine on pages 52 and 53.
FRIDAY			✓*		*Choose one of the four water aerobic programs.
SATURDAY		REST			
SUNDAY		REST			

WEEK #3

EXERCISE DAY OF THE WEEK	GYM/SPORT ACTIVITY (SEE PAGES 31–41)	WALK AND WALK/JOG (SEE PAGE 58)	WATER AEROBICS (SEE PAGE 59)	☑ CHECK WHEN COMPLETED	COMMENTS
MONDAY	✓*				*Choose a gym aerobic machine, dance class, or sport activity. Do 30 minutes.
TUESDAY (CROSS-TRAINING)					Complete the eight-exercise routine on pages 52 and 53.
WEDNESDAY			✓*		*Choose one of the four water aerobic programs.
THURSDAY (CROSS-TRAINING)					Complete the eight-exercise routine on pages 52 and 53.
FRIDAY		✓*			*Choose either program one, two, or three depending on your current fitness level.
SATURDAY		REST			
SUNDAY		REST			

WEEK #4

abdominals (abs): The muscles that support the area of the body between the chest and the pelvis.

aerobic: Needing oxygen for physical activity.

aerobic exercise: Pphysical activity that increases the intake of oxygen, and improves the cardiovascular and respiratory systems.

balance: The even distribution of weight that enables a person to remain upright and steady; also called equilibrium.

ballistic stretching: A form of stretching that uses momentum to force a muscle group or joint beyond its normal range of motion.

blood pressure: Pressure exerted against arterial walls.

body weight exercises: A type of exercise in which the weight of your body is used as resistance (example: modified push-ups).

calf muscles: The two large muscles in the back of the lower leg.

cardiovascular fitness: Another term for aerobic fitness—cardio for heart; vascular for blood vessels.

core: The muscles of the hips, pelvis, trunk, shoulders, and neck.

cramp: A sudden, involuntary, painful contraction of a muscle.

diastolic: The lower (bottom) number in a blood pressure reading that reflects pressure within arteries between heartbeats.

delayed onset muscle soreness (DOMS): A condition involving muscle overuse that usually develops a day or two after an especially demanding workout.

• **dynamic stretches:** Stretches designed to move the body through a range of motion that mimics the physical activity in which you are participating.

extension: Straightening or extending a joint or limb of the body.

fasting plasma glucose test: A measurement of glucose levels after not having anything to eat or drink (other than water) for at least eight hours before the test.

flexion: Bending a joint or limb of the body.

flexibility: The range of motion through which a joint moves.

free weights: Dumbbells, barbells, or kettlebells (examples) used in resistance training.

hamstrings: Muscles or tendons behind the back part of the upper legs.

high-impact aerobic exercise: Physical activity that results in a heart rate of approximately 80-85 percent of maximum, and in which there is a greater impact on bones and joints.

high intensity interval training (HIIT): Involves short bursts of intense activity followed by brief recovery periods

ligament: A tissue that connects bones or cartilage.

low-impact aerobic exercise: Physical activity in which there is a less-demanding cardiovascular effort and in which one foot is always in contact with the ground or surface.

maximum heart rate: The heart rate a person should not exceed for any extended length of time.

medial tibial stress syndrome: The medical term for shin splints.

metabolic equivalent (MET): A unit of measurement used to estimate the amount of oxygen used during physical activity.

mobility: the ability to move in one's environment with ease and without restriction.

muscle imbalance: refers to opposite muscle groups (biceps/triceps, for example) that are not balanced in terms of strength.

obesity: a higher level of being overweight in relation to height, sometimes defined as being 20 percent over healthy weight.

osteoarthritis (OA): a disease characterized by the degeneration of cartilage and the underlying bone.

osteopenia: Lower-than-normal bone density.

osteoporosis: A disease in which the bones become weak, brittle, and porous.

overweight: A weight that is not healthy for a person of a given height.

plantar faciitis: An inflammation of the tissue that runs along the bottom surface of the foot from the heel to the base of the toes.

pronation: The action of the feet when the ankles turn inward when walking or running (also refers to the motion of the forearm when turning the palm downward).

quadriceps: Large muscles on the upper front area of the legs.

recovery heart rate: The time it takes the heart to return to its normal resting rate after exercise.

repetition (rep): The single act of lifting or moving a part of the body against resistance.

resistance training: A form of exercise that involves movement or attempted movement against resistance (or load).

sarcopenia: Age-related loss of muscle mass and strength.

set: The number of repetitions of an exercise movement.

shin splints: An informal term for pain in the front or inner part of the lower leg.

sprain: An injury caused by forcing a joint beyond its normal range of motion.

strain: A stretched or torn muscle or tendon, informally referred to as a pulled muscle.

strength: The ability to exert force against resistance.

stress fracture: A type of broken bone in which there are small cracks often caused by repetitive application of force or overuse.

systolic: The top (upper) number in a blood pressure reading that reflects pressure within arterial walls when the heart muscle contracts.

target heart rate zone: A heart rate range of approximately 55 to 85 percent of maximum heart rate in which a person strives to train aerobically.

tendon: A tissue that connects muscles to bones and cartilage.

torso: The trunk of the body.

weight training: Also called resistance training, in which a person lifts or moves weights to gain muscle strength or endurance.

American Academy of Orthopaedic Surgeons
www.aaos.org
847-823-7186
9400 West Higgins Rd.
Rosemont, IL 60018

American Academy of Physical Medicine & Rehabilitation
www.aapmr.org
847-737-6000
9700 West Bryn Mawr Ave.
Suite 200
Rosemont, IL 60018-5701

American College of Sports Medicine
www.acsm.org
317-637-9200
401 West Michigan St.
Indianapolis, IN 46202-3233

American Council on Exercise
www.acefitness.org
888-825-3636
4851 Paramount Dr.
San Diego, CA 92123

American Heart Association
www.heart.org
800-242-8721
7272 Greenville Ave.
Dallas, TX 75231

American Orthopaedic Foot & Ankle Society
www.aofas.org
800-235-4855
9400 West Higgins Rd.
Suite 220
Rosemont, IL 60018

American Physical Therapy Association
www.apta.org/BalanceFalls/
800-999-2782
3030 Potomac Ave.
Suite 100
Alexandria, VA 22305-3085

American Podiatric Medical Association
www.apma.org
301-581-9200
9312 Old Georgetown Rd.
Bethesda, MD 20814-1621

Arthritis Foundation
www.arthritis.org
1.800.283.7800
1355 Peachtree St NE
Suite 600
Atlanta, GA 30309

Centers for Disease Control and Prevention
www.cdc.gov
800-232-4636
1600 Clifton Rd.
Atlanta, GA 30329-4027

Center for Healthy Aging
www.ncoa.org/improve-health/center-for-healthy-aging
202-479-1200
National Council on Aging
251 18th St. S
Arlington, VA 22202

National Association for
www.physicalfitness.org
518-456-1058
Health and Fitness
10 Kings Mill Ct.
Albany, NY 12205-3632

National Institute on Aging
www.nia.nih.gov
800-222-2225
31 Center Dr.
MSC 2292
Bethesda, MD 20892

National Safety Council
www.nsc.org
800-621-7615
1121 Spring Lake Dr.
Itasca, IL 60143-3201

National Strength & Conditioning Association
www.nsca.com
719-632-6722
1885 Bob Johnson Dr.
Colorado Springs, CO 80906

Office of Disease Prevention and Health Promotion
www.health.gov
email: odphpinfo@hhs.gov
U.S. Department of Health and Human Services
1101 Wootton Pkwy.
Suite LL100
Rockville, MD 20852

President's Council on Fitness, Sports & Nutrition
www.fitness.gov
240-276-9567
1101 Wootton Pkwy.
Suite 560
Rockville, MD 20852

U.S. Department of Veterans Affairs
www.patientsafety.va.gov
810 Vermont Ave., NW
Washington, DC 20571

UCLA Health System
www.uclahealth.org
310-825-0014
Cardiac and Pulmonary Rehabilitation
100 UCLA Medical Plaza
Suite 440
Los Angeles, CA 90095

YMCA of the USA
www.ymca.net
800-872-9622
101 North Wacker Dr.
Suite 1600
Chicago, IL 60606